THE AMAZING POWER OF HYPNOSIS

WHAT IT CAN DO FOR YOU

The Amazing Power of Hypnosis

WHAT IT CAN DO FOR YOU

Wesley Shrader

DOUBLEDAY & COMPANY, INC.
GARDEN CITY, NEW YORK
1976

Abridgment of letter of July 20, 1952, by Aldous Huxley in *Letters of Aldous Huxley*, edited by Grover Smith. Copyright © 1969 by Laura Huxley. Copyright © 1969 by Grover Smith. Reprinted by permission of Harper & Row, Publishers and Chatto and Windus Ltd.

Library of Congress Cataloging in Publication Data

Shrader, Wesley.
   The amazing power of hypnosis.

   Bibliography
   1. Hypnotism—Therapeutic use—Cases, clinical
reports, statistics.   I. Title.
RC495.S53   615'.8512'0926
ISBN 0-385-07088-8
Library of Congress Catalog Card Number 75-14840

To the memory of
PROFESSOR PAUL SCHUBERT

Foreword

Those who read *The Amazing Power of Hypnosis* will indeed be amazed by the breadth of human problems solved by hypnotic technique: problems of attention and concentration, problems of sexual functioning, problems of disturbed sleep. In addition to these kinds of "normal" abnormalities, the reader will find chapters on more serious problems such as alcoholism and stuttering. These problems plaguing large segments of humanity are familiar ones. Within the covers of this book symptoms become human dilemmas. Persons suffering under their burden are real people, and their relationship with Wesley Shrader are equally real and intimate.

There is no better way of understanding the technique of hypnotherapy than to study Dr. Shrader's detailed account of his work with his patients. What does such a study reveal? Two main points strike me as pre-eminent: first, that the technique of hypnotherapy, like that of all psychotherapy, is dependent upon the mutual participation of patient and therapist; second, the solutions attained in hypnotherapy are primarily dependent upon the creative and innovative response of the therapist, and certainly not his reliance upon either frozen formula or authoritarian charisma.

If these two simple truths had been available during the last seventy or eighty years, the course of psychotherapy would have been quite different. Indeed, the current upsurge of interest in hypnosis is not a novel one. One cannot talk about hypnosis without making reference to its "boom and bust" history. We know why boom, but why bust? The explanation is simple: having discovered the process of hypnosis, we hoped to dispense it by formula. However, it is one thing to duplicate the tricks of the stage hypnotist, and quite a different thing to relate to human problems. One can make an analogy to medicine and suggest that if we place our hope in hypnosis as a new antibiotic, which could be injected to cure a disease, we are disappointed. On the other hand, if hypnosis is viewed as a surgical technique, we can appreciate the fact that success or failure of any particular application depends upon the specific adaptation of a complex technology, by a competent expert, to a wide range of contingencies.

Wesley Shrader's work is exactly this kind of pioneering, front-line work. From this volume the layman may find a better insight into one of his personal problems or a problem of someone around him. Professionals can learn about the relationship of improvisational responses to involvement with the patient-as-person. The range of techniques demonstrated is very broad, particularly techniques associated with response change.

I cannot conclude these remarks without referring to the single most impressive quality of this book; namely, its simple, direct concern for the person. In so doing, Dr. Shrader, as counselor and as healer, conveys by example the primary axiom of every psychotherapist: that patients are persons estranged from community and that "symptoms" are cries for help.

ANTHONY B. GABRIELE, Ph.D.

Preface

Public interest in hypnosis is far greater today than it was ten years ago, and there is also a growing interest on the part of physicians, dentists, psychiatrists, psychoanalysts, and counselors to know more about this amazing power. For more than a quarter of a century I have practiced hypnosis in connection with my counseling ministry. Because of rejection in certain academic and church circles, I did so as quietly as possible.

However, for the past ten years, I have virtually hung out a shingle and have devoted as much time to this work as possible. During this period I continued study and research, and, of course, I worked with many more people with serious problems than ever before. I have seen changes take place in my own personality, especially in being relaxed while living in a pressure cooker (New York) and being able to handle a variety of complicated responsibilities.

Instead of attempting a "handbook" to assist would-be hypnotists "to learn how to do it," I have described the lives of twenty-six people and have shown how each was aided by hypnosis. Every account in this book is true, the people are real, and their problems are real. For obvious reasons, in certain instances, names and places have been changed. I hope that readers with similar problems will read the stories and attempt to identify with one or more of them.

In recounting these stories I have presented the variety of emphases in the range of hypnotic induction, such as the various levels one may reach and how these levels are detected. Also important areas of the hypnotic field are described. These include regression, amnesia, anesthesia, phobias, hallucination, relaxation, and loss of tension.

I am grateful to the hundreds of people with whom I have worked during these many years, but most of all I am indebted to the members of my congregation who share with me the conviction that hypnosis is none other than the power of God working through receptive persons.

WESLEY SHRADER
New York City

Contents

THE AMAZING POWER OF HYPNOSIS

WHAT IT CAN DO FOR YOU

I

Hypnosis and the Common Phobia

It was a long, long time ago, but just the same I shall never forget the look on Helen's face when I told her that I had done all I could to help her. She asked, "Do you think I'll be this way forever?"

The place was Lexington, Kentucky; I was recently graduated from the seminary, where I absorbed biblical studies, theology, and a rather heavy dose of psychology. Courses in Pastoral Care or Pastoral Psychology were becoming quite the thing in seminaries about that time. I had seen Helen a number of times in counseling sessions. She was in her forties, was obese, and talked with a strange type of wheezing. But obesity and wheezing were not the problem she was most concerned about. She was afraid to ride on a railroad train, the most prevalent form of travel in those days. Besides, her husband worked for the railroad, which meant she could ride the trains virtually free of charge. But she was blocked, dead center. She could not set foot in a railroad coach. In conversation I had taken her over the familiar ground which I had been taught. Why was Helen afraid to ride trains? Had she been frightened by a train in her childhood? Had any catastrophe happened to anyone in her family in connection with trains? What about dreams? Could she remember having nightmares about trains? So, on and on we went.

Then I turned to religion with a little "positive thinking" thrown in. I prayed with her at the end of each session and gave her a Bible verse to remember and repeat each morning and evening. It was a beautiful verse, "Perfect love casts out fear."

As the days went by, Helen became more frightened than when I first began to see her. There was no practicing psychiatrist in Lexington at the time to whom I could refer her. However, as she was extremely religious and held to the views of the day, she would not have gone to a psychiatrist. So when she asked, "Do you think I'll be this way forever?" I gave her the best answer I could think of: "I doubt that you'll be this way forever. *Time* does wonders; it heals us when all else fails." She left my office. Three months later she and her husband moved to Nashville, Tennessee. I have had no word from Helen since, but my guess is, if she is alive, and in spite of the assurance I gave her, she is still afraid to ride on trains.

Was it coincidence or Providence that my close friend John Handy, professor of psychology at the University of Kentucky, hit me with a straightforward question: "Wes, do you know anything about hypnosis?" We were eating lunch in the university cafeteria. I put my fork down, looked at him with some irritation, and said, "I know absolutely nothing about hypnosis, and furthermore, I would not give the subject a second thought."

As was the case with my psychology friend, I cut my teeth on Freud, Adler, Jung, Sullivan, Theodor Reik, Otto Rank, Fenichel, Horney, etc. None of these "greats" placed much stock in hypnosis. Freud, I remember reading, tried it and in disgust gave it up. I expressed the latter sentiment to John Handy.

He responded with some heat. "You're dead wrong about Freud. He retained an interest in hypnosis until he died." Before I could reply to his comment, he continued, "You see a remarkable number of people in counseling situations. If you mastered the art of hypnotic induction and application, I am sure you could help a larger number of them."

What brought on this conversation was that I had told my psychologist friend the story of Helen and her fear of trains. "John," I said, "I respect you and your professionalism. However, I have no interest in, no faith in, hypnosis. To me it is quackery, nothing more or less."

He laughed and said, "Do me a favor. Go to the library, take out two books: Clark Hull's *Hypnosis and Suggestibility* and Forel's *Hypnotism.*"

I brushed him off, even as I have since been brushed off many times with: "I may get around to it one of these days."

A month or so later, I was in the library and the professor's suggestion about Hull and Forel strangely came to me. But stronger still was the image of Helen and my inability to help her.

I was amazed at the amount of material in the stacks on "Hypnosis"; some of the authors I recognized and some were unknown to me. I checked out Hull and Forel, and from that day to this I have been hooked on the power of hypnosis.

John Handy was more than pleased when he saw my enthusiasm. He invited me to join a small group of graduate students and one other professor. He was the leader of the group, which met once each week; of course, without college credit. The primary purpose was research and experimentation. Research, at the time I joined the group, was concerned with amnesia hypnosis, but later advanced to regression, anesthesia, and phobias. It was several years before I agreed to hypnotize anyone outside of this group. I found that the common phobia was one of the easiest to deal with. *I am convinced that with hypnosis I could have aided Helen and her fear of trains.*

For this chapter I have chosen six people, each with his own deep-seated fear. These have been selected from dozens of people who suffered from similar complaints. There are rational fears which sane people possess and which enable them to survive in our kind of world. A child must be taught early in life to have proper respect for, and even a fear of, an open fire. An elderly person fears to walk certain streets in New York after dark. These are not irrational feelings; they are necessary to survival. On the other hand, when a woman of twenty-five is frightened out of her wits by a feather, or being alone in a room with the door closed, she is possessed of an irrational fear. This is what we mean by a phobia.

1. The Football Player—Fear of Flying

Jack Daly sat across the room from me, a living picture in livid color of a person who was at that moment facing imminent danger. He was twenty-one years of age, weighed 235 pounds, and was the star fullback on the university football team. The team was leaving the next day for a cross-country destination to play one of its important games.

Jack's voice quavered as he said, "I don't know what in the hell is wrong with me. When I was a freshman we played a short schedule, and *only one plane trip*. I had never been on a plane before. As the time of departure got nearer, I grew apprehensive, but told no one about how I felt. I managed to hold myself together and play reasonably well."

"What about your sophomore year? Did you continue about the same or has the fear increased?"

His hands were wet with sweat, and I could tell that his pulse rate had increased as he recounted the agony he endured in his sophomore year. "Last year was pain, it was hell, just thinking about the next trip, and then enduring it. Drinking liquor was too obvious. I would have been suspended immediately. However, I tried sleeping pills and tranquilizers . . . but just once! They zonked me out. I was so flat for the game that the coach took me out and said, 'Jack, you're too damn sick to be on that field. Go to the clubhouse and see the trainer.' "

Feeling ashamed, he had kept his phobia secret. He had made up a story to the doctor who had given him the prescription for the pills. Now he was confronted with flying across country for the first game of his junior year. Bigger, stronger, and more bullish than ever, he was a contrast in brute strength and hand-sweating terror, like a child afraid of the dark.

I asked Jack to sit back in the chair, place his hands loosely on his thighs, close his eyes for about a minute, concentrating on one subject, perhaps a flickering candle or a pleasant scene. I explained to him that as he took five deep breaths on my counting he would begin to feel the tension leave his body. I then gave suggestions concerning muscular relaxation. "From head to toe, every muscle in your body is now beginning to feel relaxed." Next came the suggestions concerning the loss of hypertension. "Hypertension," I said, "is nothing more than excessive emotional energy which builds up within you. As this emotion begins to leave your body, you may feel the tip of your fingers or your toes begin to tingle." Then Jack entered what I call the period of "breathing of sleep," breath a little heavier and more rhythmic. "This is the breathing of sleep," I repeated six or eight times. "Now you are feeling drowsy and drowsier, sleepy and sleepier." By the time we reached this point, I was convinced that Jack was a responsive hypnotic subject. The subconscious part of his mind began to take over. Suggestions relating to *application* were now in order. "Jack, tomorrow as you board that plane, let me describe how you will feel. The overpowering feeling will be one of boredom. Few people enjoy riding in a plane for five or six hours at a time. So you will join most of us and become just bored. The thought of fear of flying will not once enter your mind. You will be amazed to discover that you forgot to be afraid . . . really forgot it." Success with Jack was somewhat easier because he had never suffered nausea with his fear. I then suggested, "Sit back, squirm in your seat if you feel like it, but above all eat everything that the stewardess brings you and more if you can get it! Eating will be the most enjoyable part of the trip." His love of food and being able to eat and retain it would reinforce the suggestion that he would forget to be afraid. Many of these charter planes that carry athletes are loaded with food many times superior to coach food.

I gave the count of five and said, "When the last count is reached, you will open your eyes, your mind will be bright and clear, but above all you will remain in this relaxed condition."

I did something with Jack Daly that I do with nearly all phobic cases as well as with many others. With a little patience and strong motivation a subject can be taught self-induction in one or two sessions. Self-induction has five steps:

1. Eyes-closed concentration on a single object for about sixty seconds.
2. Three to five deep breaths.
3. Pleasant suggestions concerning limpness of the body, limb by limb.
4. A reminder that muscular relaxation, release of tension, and lowering the anxiety level are being experienced.
5. A positive suggestion, without referring to the specific fear, such as "You may be bored with the trip, but you will enjoy the food more than ever."

During the past several years I have discovered that self-hypnosis is more effective with most (not all) people if they stand outside of themselves and use the word "you" instead of "I." *Your* head is becoming heavier, *your* eyelids are becoming heavier. *You* are becoming drowsy. And so forth. I do not know yet why this is more effective. I only know that it is so, and that I myself use this method each day for simple relaxation and loss of tension.

Jack came to see me the next week. He was in no need of another hypnotic session. He exclaimed, "The trip *was* a bore, but the food was great, the stewardesses were knockouts—I dated one after the game. . . ." He paused and was serious for a moment. "I forgot to be afraid; I really did. I really forgot to be afraid."

Jack continued daily with his exercises in self-induction, experimenting here and there. One day he asked me, "This stuff is spooky. . . . Is there any danger in my doing it every day?"

I replied, "None whatsoever; nothing but good will come from it."

2. The Housewife—Fear of Choking

I explained in the previous section that a phobia is an *irrational* fear. The more we intellectualize the irrationality of such a fear, the worse we suffer. I could have spent days with Jack piling up argument after argument which would demonstrate the foolishness in refusing to ride in a plane: "Planes are the safest mode of transportation—many times safer than riding in an automobile or on trains." I could have pointed out that more serious accidents occur in homes and apartments than anywhere else. But when one is dealing with an irrational condition, intellectualizing, moralizing, arguing will not solve the problem.

Hypnosis is not totally irrational, though there is an irrational, primal element in it. The irrational element is the same as it is with the atom. Do we really know what an atom is? Are we completely satisfied and convinced when we are told that "an atom is the smallest amount of an element that is capable of existence." This statement has little meaning to the average person; it has less for the scientist. He sees the atom in the context of a vast system of imponderables. However, we have learned many ways to harness the atom for good and ill. So it is with hypnosis. How is it that one man sitting in a chair, and simply talking to a person opposite him, creates within that person conditions which have no natural explanation? As the hands can be made hot or cold, heavy or light, so can blood pressure be brought down or up, pulse rate can be slowed or the rate can become faster. With the atom and electricity, total explanations elude us; so it is with hypnosis. There is one difference: the element of danger in hypnosis is virtually lacking, whereas with the atom and with electricity the element of immense danger is ever present.

Tamara, a woman of forty-six, was possessed of an irrational phobia. She was afraid to eat solid food. Two years prior to her seeing me, she choked on a fishbone and almost suffocated. In this instance we think we know the "why" of her condition. The cause of her not eating solid food for nearly two years was the fact that she had choked on a fishbone. However, a close observer would not accept this explanation as final. Tamara had entered menopause at about age forty-three, and though many women today breeze through this condition, she, from the beginning, was having a difficult time. I listened for about an hour to her story of not being able to eat good solid food, of choking on the fishbone, and of her many symptoms which she associated with menopause.

She cried, "Unless I can get help somewhere I'll lose my mind."

I replied, "Suppose there was a pill or an injection which would help you change your life style. Instead of being a highly nervous person, you would know what it is to be relaxed and at ease. You would feel the loss of hypertension; you would know what it means to manage your anxiety level. Just suppose—"

She interrupted me with a shout. "But there isn't any such pill and you know it."

"That's correct. No pill, no injection, no knife can do the trick for you. *You* must be changed."

"How will my being changed, becoming relaxed and whatever else you said, get me over the fear of eating and being choked to death?"

"Hypnosis can give you two things: a bright, clear mind and a relaxed body. Once you become that kind of person, your fear will vanish."

She looked at me wide-eyed with unbelief.

"Think it over for a week. If by then you believe what I just said about the power of hypnosis, call me for an appointment. I would like very much to help you."

Tamara was in my office one week from that day. Tense, hostile, self-pitying, but somewhat humble, she said, "I am ready."

So we began the first hypnotic session. She was medium responsive, sufficiently so to experience total loss of tension. I went through a similar type of induction with Tamara as I did with Jack Daly. However, Jack had to fly the next day. With Tamara I could take more time.

Bringing her out of the trance, I said, "Take your time . . . nobody is in a hurry."

She was silent for several minutes, and then softly said, "Never in my life have I ever felt so relaxed. . . . I heard everything you said. You didn't mention anything about being able to eat a good meal."

"We'll get to that sooner or later."

For the first time since I had known her—which was about three years—I saw Tamara smile. She left my office with peace of mind and said, "I do feel better."

The second session we achieved a greater degree of relaxation. Deep vertical lines had formed down the bridge of her nose. These disappeared! It was an excellent sign.

While she was still under hypnosis, I said, "Tonight, you will eat and you will eat with pleasure anything you desire." She had lost about thirty pounds during her season of irrational fear. She could gain at least fifteen or twenty pounds and be none the worse. When she was still under the hypnotic trance, I said to her, "Only one additional suggestion. Your food will taste so good tonight that you must guard against stuffing or glutting. Eat just enough to satisfy your desire."

She called me about ten o'clock that night. "I couldn't wait," she said. "I ate my first satisfying meal in nearly two years. May I make an appointment to see you again?"

Another week went by. She entered my office obviously less tense. She was a person who was achieving a new life style, a sense of well-being.

"Today," I said, "you will hypnotize yourself."

"How in the world?"

"First, I will hypnotize you. You'll achieve the greatest degree of relaxation. I will then give the suggestion that you will become a master of self-hypnosis."

She achieved her hypnotic state easily. I made the suggestion concerning self-hypnosis. Then I brought her out of the trance with her mind bright and clear and her body strong but relaxed.

After a few minutes I said, "Now close your eyes and begin the self-induction." I was the coach, she was the eager learner.

She went through the paces. Her head became heavy, her body relaxed, all anxiety disappeared. Aloud she made the suggestion: "You are beginning to experience a sense of well-being, you will learn to enjoy the good things of life, including food."

The irrational fear of choking disappeared, but what was more amazing, a lovely personality began to develop. Tamara, hostile and self-pitying, became a beautiful person interested in the welfare of others as well as herself.

3. The Artist—Fear of Going Out

I always considered agoraphobia to be one of the rarest phobias among us until I moved to New York eight years ago. But it is not rare; more people suffer from it with varying degrees of intensity than I suspected. Agoraphobia is the panic which attacks the subject as he contemplates leaving, or as he actually begins to leave, the womb of his secure surroundings. Though I do not pretend that my figures are definitive, I have found more men with this fear than women. Even if you have never been so cursed, you can, with a little imagination, begin to appreciate the difficulties this particular defect has for one so gripped. It often means giving up employment and going on welfare as well as sacrificing all social life. Such a victim is literally housebound.

Victor and Dean were brothers who lived on Staten Island, one of the five boroughs of New York. It is reached by the famous Staten Island ferry or now by the Verrazano Bridge from Brooklyn. I much prefer working with subjects on my home base. One should be able to hold a hypnotic conversation almost anywhere, but I prefer my own office.

Victor was the older of the two brothers, about forty-five. He worked for a large bank on Wall Street, was strong, healthy, not married, and spent most of his spare time looking after and caring for Dean, the younger brother. Dean, thirty-eight, was a first-rate artist who could function well so long as he confined himself to the family home. He had not left the house—it is more accurate to say he had not left the grounds of the house—since the funeral of his mother and father five years before. The parents had been killed together in an automobile accident. In the spring and fall he would walk around the spacious yard and enjoy the beauties of nature, or he would just sit quietly and meditate in the garden.

I had known Victor a number of years, but had never met Dean. One day Victor came by my office at the noon hour, found me free, and we enjoyed renewing an old friendship which dated back to the years I lived in New Haven, Connecticut. He told me about his brother's pathetic condition and finally said, "Would you come over to the house and see him?"

I laughed and said, "I rarely make hypnotic house calls."

He said seriously, "I believe you can help Dean. He has agreed to try hypnosis, but he can't leave the house." The parents had left their estate and small fortune to the two brothers. There was no difficulty getting barbers, dentists, physicians, and others to make house calls. My friendship with Victor and also the challenge of working with someone suffering from agoraphobia led to my consent to go to Staten Island, meet the brother, and give whatever help possible. Agoraphobia does not respond to therapy easily. It is claustrophobia (fear of small enclosed places) drawn on a large canvas. But the primary difficulty in helping such a subject is his *innate resistance* to receiving help from anyone.

On a lovely Saturday afternoon in early October, Victor picked me up in his limousine. We crossed the Brooklyn Bridge, made our way to the Verrazano Bridge, and within a relatively short time were on Staten Island at Victor's estate.

Dean was in the garden as we drove up. He came to the front of the surrounding fence and met us. I was introduced. "This is Wesley Shrader, whom I met in New Haven a number of years ago."

Dean was a handsome young man, slightly effeminate, but with a charming smile. As he shook my hand he said, "I feel as if I've known you for years. Victor has—"

Victor interrupted with a laugh. "Years ago Wesley helped me break a three-pack-a-day cigarette habit. That makes him something of a miracle man!"

We enjoyed tea, some marvelous fluffy shell cakes served by the manservant of the house, called Jake. Jake had been the family chauffeur for years. After a while Victor excused himself and said, "I'll let you two talk. Jake has asked me to pick up several things at the supermarket and bakery. I'll be back in about forty minutes."

I studied Dean carefully. He was as well put together as anyone I had met in a long time. No weight problem, no money problems, a successful career in art. He was associated with a large gallery on upper Madison Avenue. The gallery had no difficulty in moving his products of labor of love. Dean showed me his studio. He indicated that it was his custom to work on four or five pictures at a time. Each picture received his attention depending upon his mood and also on the type of light available.

At last, moving from one room of the great house to another, we came to a cozy reading room with comfortable chairs.

Dean broke the ice. His voice was firm, his charming features unchanged. "You may think you're here because Victor pressured me into seeing you. That's not true. I have checked out your work not only with people you have worked with but also several psychoanalysts and psychiatrists. I want to be helped. I must overcome this fanatical fear of leaving the grounds."

"I would not have come for a hypnotic session if *you* had not wanted me. I would have come for a visit with Victor and you, but not for hypnosis. With hypnosis, 'you gotta believe.'"

"Have you worked before with people suffering from this problem?"

"Several."

"Help any?"

"All who were responsive to the hypnotic procedure were helped. Those who did not trust me or felt that hypnosis was a game or nonsense were not helped." I then described the procedure with two other people with whom I had recently worked, a woman and a man, both about Dean's age. "These people found releas' from panic. They are now well, functioning, and happy. I asked each of them permission to give you their names and numbers. Perhaps you might call one or both of these people. Furthermore, if it suits you, we might have a group discussion here at your home."

"Something like a meeting of 'Phobia Anonymous.'"

"Precisely," I said in good humor.

Next week my two friends, Dean, and I met in the great house on Staten Island. After an easy round of introductions, we began the meeting in the same way as an AA meeting.

Arlene, the recovered agoraphobiac, began with a brief recital of her difficulty and how she came to my office with fear and trembling. She explained our interview and in detail described the soothing effect the hypnotic process had on her strained emotions. At the end of her fifth session she flew to California with her husband for business and vacation.

Arlene had an excellent sense of humor and interlaced her story with comedic punch lines. Her condition had not been as severe as Dean's. At the time she first saw me, she could leave her apartment but could not leave Manhattan and could not ride buses and subways.

Merle, a single man in his early forties, had a condition almost as serious as Dean's. He lived with his mother on the Upper East Side. He could leave the apartment for a few minutes, so long as his mother escorted him. But "going out" to a department store, the dentist, the theater was virtually impossible. He came to my office in pain and recounted his experience in excellent diction, but with little humor. However, his experience with hypnosis had been miraculous. Within a few weeks he returned to an executive position in his late father's business and was on the job virtually every day.

I studied Dean carefully as these stories were presented. His handsome face became tense as he recounted his experience with agoraphobia. He had not been beyond the bounds of the estate since returning from his parents' funeral. His gallery was on upper Madison Avenue in Manhattan, and he wanted very much to keep up with his contemporaries in the world of art, his first love. He said that he cared little about traveling abroad or around the United States; however, he did want very much to be able to go from Staten Island to Manhattan.

After this mini-encounter session, I asked Arlene and Merle to join Victor on the terrace. Victor was waiting for them with cocktails. After they left the room I asked Dean, "Are you ready for your first hypnotic session?"

He replied, "Yes, I'm looking forward to it."

Dean was easily inducted. The smile which he sometimes forced disappeared from his face. Within minutes he was a picture of relief. I gave him the following posthypnotic suggestion: "Dean, you are now totally relaxed; anxiety has disappeared; the subconscious part of your mind has taken over. From here on, it does not matter whether you remember what I say. Tomorrow evening about seven o'clock, just about when all the lights in Manhattan have been turned on, you and Victor will make the trip to Manhattan. *But not in the car.* You will park the car at the dock, board the Staten Island ferry, and take the ride to Manhattan." (The ride lasts about twenty-five minutes.) "Arlene, Merle, and I will be on the other side to meet the ferry. Then we'll go to one of the best restaurants in New York, atop a beautiful skyscraper. There we shall eat and drink, but most of all we shall enjoy each other's company as well as the view of the lighted city. . . . Do you fully understand?"

"Yes," he said, "I understand."

I replied, "The spirit in which you do this is important. Beginning this very moment, there must be created deep within your emotional life an eagerness for the experience. Something like a performer looking forward to opening night on Broadway . . . eagerness, anticipation, exhilaration."

The session was soon over.

Dean said, "My God, what an experience. I feel loose and limp."

"Do you remember what I said about tomorrow night?"

He paused for several minutes, a curious smile-frown crossed his face. He said, "I remember everything but your final words."

"It doesn't matter. The suggestion will come to you as we review it with the others."

"Wait . . . wait just a minute," he said slowly. "I do remember. You said that Victor and I were to go to Manhattan on the ferry. Something I have not done in years. How I loved it when I was a

kid! You will meet us at the other side. . . . Arlene and Merle will
be with you and we'll have a night on the town!"

"Exactly."

One hypnotic session with Dean was sufficient. However, it was
the prior buildup that prepared him for recovery. At my suggestion,
these three people met in each other's apartments once a week for
several months. Dean each time made the trip to Manhattan. The
first couple of times he was accompanied by his brother. At last he
said, "I would like to go alone."

When he reached that stage he was no longer a prisoner of the irrational fear that had dominated his life for more than five years.

4. The Model—Fear of Gaining Weight

Candy called me early on a Monday morning. She was in tears.
Her physician had recommended that she see me. "What is the nature of your problem?" I asked.

"Weight," she answered.

Obesity has the same orientation as alcoholism. Eating is so normal, so very much a part of our culture that until one becomes
gross, no one pays too much attention to it.

Candy came in the early part of the following week. I had made a
few notes on our telephone conversation. They read: "Candy
L. . . . works as model . . . overweight . . . out-of-control eating
. . . age bracket, under thirty," and included the name of her family physician.

At 9 A.M. she came into my office. There have been a few
times when my secretary and I get appointments confused. She will
schedule a person for one hour and I will schedule another for the
same hour. It hasn't happened often, but I must admit *it has happened*. The young lady standing before me nervously put out her
hand and said, "My name is Candy. . . . I called you last week for
an appointment."

Rarely have I been at a loss for words in the counseling room. I
seriously doubt that there has been an experience which I have not
been introduced to. Everything from having to wrestle a knife away
from a female paranoiac who had come to kill me because I had or-

ganized an underworld gang to silence her, to every type of sexual aberration. As this tense, strained young woman stood in my presence, I was at a loss for words.

Thinking of nothing better to say, I said, "Please have a seat on the couch."

She sat, gingerly, carefully, fearfully.

I saw no reason to beat about the bush. "You called about being overweight, an uncontrolled eater. You appear everything else but a person struggling with obesity."

"But I am . . . that's my problem."

I asked her a few questions for the record. She was under thirty, she was 5 feet 6 inches, she weighed 112 pounds and had held this weight since adolescence. She worked as a model and as an actress in TV commercials. She obviously was making a good living.

"Here's the way I control my weight," she said.

I nodded.

"For *breakfast*, I have one cup of black coffee, with a couple of cigarettes. . . . *Lunch*, I eat salad with low-calorie dressing. I vary this; the day I do not eat a salad I will eat an apple or orange for lunch. . . . At the *evening meal*, I am hungry. I usually eat seafood, vegetables, another salad, and a couple of glasses of wine, no bread, no potatoes, no sweets."

"Anything to drink before the evening meal?" I asked.

"Most of the time a single or double scotch."

"What about between-meals and late-night snacks?"

"I never eat between meals and never late at night."

"From what you have said, you are consuming approximately four hundred calories a day in food and two or three hundred in liquor, a total of about seven hundred calories a day."

"That's about what I figure."

"The manner in which you are balancing these daily diets, beginning with coffee and cigarettes in the morning, will eventually be disastrous to your health."

She said, "That's right. . . . I'm a wreck. I have a great agent, or I would never get a job. . . . I'm getting weaker and weaker. . . . I don't know how much longer I can keep going."

"Well, for one thing you can begin by eating more nutritious food."

"I didn't finish telling the whole story. . . . It's so embarrassing."

"Go ahead; take it easy," I said.

"It's like this. As quickly as I have had the last bite or the last drink, if I'm eating in a restaurant with a date, I go to the ladies' room—if I'm in my apartment, I go to the bathroom—and then I push my finger down my throat and vomit until I disgorge everything I had to eat for the evening meal."

Sitting before me was a nervous, out-of-control young woman who was not suffering from obesity or overeating. Her problem had little to do with eating. She was in the "Phobic Family," and was literally committing slow suicide with an irrational fear—the fear of food and the fear of becoming overweight.

"How do you feel about hypnosis?"

"I know nothing about . . . am fearful of it."

"Why did you call me?"

"Dr. K. said that I should see you. . . . He's done all he can for me."

"Are you willing to try a first session?" I asked.

Shakily she said, "Yes, I'm willing."

As I have indicated, the variety of phobias yield to a happy conclusion in the vast majority of instances. If the person has a minimum of faith in the process, a trustful attitude toward the operator, and is reasonably cooperative, as was Dean in the last section, good and permanent results are more often than not obtained.

Candy was prepared to go through a hypnotic process, whatever that meant. Her physician said that it had worked for several of his patients.

I said, "Sit on the couch as comfortably as possible. Close your eyes and keep them closed until I tell you to open them. Now take five deep breaths." She was still rigid and uptight.

From this point I gave suggestions about the various parts of the body becoming more and more relaxed, emotional tension being eased, anxiety level lowered. I suggested that she would begin to experience soothing feelings of drowsiness. Then I began with several exercises, each designed to increase the hypnotic depth. I started with the eyelids. "Open your eyes on the count of one, close them on two. You will find that your eyelids have become heavy, extremely heavy. Do not strain, disregard the count if you feel extreme heaviness in the eyelids." She opened her eyes with the greatest ease. There was no heaviness. I asked her to clasp her hands together tightly. "You will find they are stuck. When I get to the count of three, your hands will be stuck, you cannot pull them apart. . . . One, two, three." She pulled her hands apart with no effort.

I had assumed a permissive attitude toward Candy. My voice was as soothing as possible. I kept repeating suggestions. My voice became rhythmic, then monotonous. I then assumed more of an authoritarian role and resorted to one more exercise. A spot on either hand of a subject can be made numb for a few minutes merely by touching it and counting. This is known as the "analgesic exercise"; she would feel no pain when I pinched the skin of the numbed spot. I repeated this suggestion several times. Then I said more strongly, "I shall pinch the skin, you will feel nothing."

I pinched.

Candy yelled, "That hurt . . . that really hurt."

I suggested that she rest for a few moments. Then I said, "You may open your eyes, tension will be gone, and you will feel relaxed."

She opened her eyes. "I don't feel relaxed. I'm scared. . . . I know I shall get as fat as a goddamn horse."

Approximately 10 per cent of the population cannot be hypnotized. Candy, in her condition, was non-hypnotizable. It is possible that someone else could help her with hypnosis, but I seriously doubt it.

Before leaving the office, she said triumphantly, "I knew you could not hypnotize me. I don't trust men, and I certainly do not intend to give up my will to anyone."

"Why did you waste your time coming here?"

"My doctor told me to come . . . but I don't trust him either."

"Why are you so suspicious of everyone?" I asked.

"Not everyone . . . just men. Can't you see how beautiful I am? Men cannot resist me. They'll do anything to get to my body."

I am sorry I made the following comment, but all of us, I suppose, say things that would be better left unsaid. "Beautiful women I see every day, but I do not consider you one of them. Your face is tense, your body is strained, and there is little strength left in you. . . ."

The words were like bullets entering her body.

She walked toward the door and started to speak, but held back. "Please," I said, "see someone before it is too late."

Candy collapsed on set several weeks after our encounter. As I write these words, she is receiving institutional care.

5. The Opera Singer—Fear of Auditioning

Mr. Theodore Sieh is on my church staff. He is the producer and artistic director of the Bel Canto Opera and has been of invaluable help to me in a variety of ways, but nowhere more helpfully than when I work with a singer who has gone out of control.

Bel Canto Opera was recently headlined in a story concerning New York's thirty-seven off-Lincoln Center opera companies. The New York *Times* rated Bel Canto one of the three best of these smaller companies. The opera has had a permanent home in our parish house since 1969. During that time, Mr. Sieh, whose musical background is impressive, has auditioned more than a thousand voices. The company has used approximately six hundred of these singers, some of whom are now performing in Germany, Italy, Spain, and various parts of this country.

Carlotta was an opera singer, financially well off, but she was in serious trouble. Here was a lovely dramatic soprano who could not stand the thought of auditioning. In recent months she had been turned down by two or three directors. Carlotta was in her late thirties, had an established reputation, and had sung for about ten years in large opera houses in Europe. She had returned to the States three years prior to my seeing her. When she entered the foyer of the parish house, she was amazed to see several striking pictures, scenes of operas which had been done by Bel Canto in recent weeks.

Her first words were, "What is an opera company doing in a church?"

I replied, "When I save an opera singer, I save a soul."

Both of us laughed easily, and then formally introduced ourselves to each other. She, like most opera people in the city, had heard of Bel Canto, but she did not associate the company with my work.

Carlotta was obviously "high strung," ambitious, and humiliated because she could not get work. "I always kill myself at the audition," she cried.

Her failure at her chosen profession during the past three years sent her toward the bottle and toward innumerable men. During our preliminary discussion, I advised her that alcohol in large doses restricts the throat as much as any other drug, and by experience she should know this.

She knew it.

Concerning men, she must determine her own needs and preferences. Since there appeared to be no guilt in these multiple relations, there is little that I had to say, except to mention what a wonderful thing it would be if she could find a man with whom she could enjoy an enduring relationship in which each would contribute strength and encouragement to the other.

"There are no such men in New York," she said dogmatically, "only homosexuals, whom I despise, and married men . . . whom I like."

"You appear to have that part of your life settled."

"Settled," she said.

I later learned that Carlotta's trouble with auditioning began a few weeks after her return from Europe. She was madly in love with a conductor of a New York opera company whose name is much more famous than Bel Canto! They had an affair in Germany. At his request she went with him to Italy and further, at his request, she sang a stand-in lead role in *Tosca* in Greece. It was this particular conductor who had been responsible for her coming back to the States. He had not planned it that way. Waiting for him in the States, after his two-month tour abroad, was a wife and three young children.

One day Carlotta showed up in New York. She contacted an artistic director hoping for an opportunity to get a role in *Tosca*. The conductor of this opera was her lover *fatal* in Europe. She sent her impressive résumé and picture to the director and indicated that she had sung the role of Tosca in Europe for the maestro.

She had attempted to telephone the conductor, but he could not be reached. She wrote several notes, stating she was in the city and giving the address of her apartment and her telephone number. There were no answers. However, the director invited her to audition on a certain late afternoon. There was a fairly large gathering of people in the recital hall that day. One after another, singers went to the stage and did their thing. Several were asked by the director to sing more than one aria. He indicated to several others that they would be called back.

At last, as Carlotta told the story, it was her turn to sing. She mounted the stage and with confidence and commanding presence she sang a notable aria from *Tosca.* As the director approached her she was positive that he was about to offer her a "call-back." She had not noticed the presence of the conductor, who had been hidden in the shadows on the extreme left of the hall. As the director approached Carlotta, so did the conductor. The director started to speak, but the conductor cut him off. "This performance [meaning Carlotta's] is precisely what we are to avoid . . . amateurish in every way."

The director started to speak, but the conductor silenced him. "Amateurish and over the hill." Carlotta was stunned by his words and so were several singers standing near enough to hear his raised voice. She ran hysterically from the recital hall and had since been seeing a psychiatrist.

It was a brutal experience. Carlotta could have been damaged permanently. Since then she had attempted several auditions—all of them complete failures. "Perhaps," she said slowly, wiping tears from her eyes, "I am over the hill."

The first session with Carlotta was taken up with her love story and her interpretation of her inability to stand before an audience or a critic and sing. Before she left, I said, "Are you ready for a hypnotic session?"

She replied, "Dr. L. thinks it may help me. I'm ready."

She came in a few days later for the introduction to hypnosis. I explained to her that there was both simplicity and mystery in hypnosis. "*Induction* means that you move from a fully conscious state to trancelike state. You will hear all that I say, you will remember most of what is said, you are not under my power, any word or suggestion which would increase anxiety would destroy the relaxed state you may have reached." I further explained that when a subject can open his eyes and retain the hypnotic state and when he is able to speak and the trance is not broken, this is an indication that the subject is extremely responsive.

Carlotta proved to be a responsive subject. Relaxation, loss of tension, and contact with the subconscious was made. Slowly I said, "Carlotta, open your eyes. Blink the lids when necessary, remain as comfortable as possible." She opened her eyes. The trance was deepened rather than being broken.

"Now I will take you by the arm and help you to stand."

With my assistance she stood. "Hold your head up straight, assume the position you take on stage when you are singing a favorite aria."

Usually, under hypnosis, the body becomes limp, the head heavy, and the voice becomes soft and low. I was now making suggestions which contradicted all of these characteristics. "When I give the signal, you will continue to stand erect, look at me or to any part of the room, open your mouth and sing . . . sing a portion of one of your favorite and familiar arias."

She sang. I have never heard a more dramatic voice. When she finished, I took her arm and assisted her to a position on the couch.

"Carlotta, the aria you sang was beautiful; your voice was strong and clear. Tomorrow when you return you will audition for Mr. Theodore Sieh, the artistic director of Bel Canto Opera."

She smiled confidently.

"Do you understand?" I asked.

"I understand."

Within seconds the session was over. Carlotta was most expressive as she said, "My God, I remember everything. . . . I sang."

"Do you remember what I said about tomorrow?"

"Certainly. I am to sing for Mr. Sieh."

"Do you know Mr. Sieh?"

"I have never met him but I know him by reputation. It will be a privilege to sing for him."

After she left I told Theodore Sieh a little bit about her traumatic experience with her first audition in the United States and that I would like for him to hear her the next day.

He asked, "How do you think she'll do? . . . Will she get through it?"

"She'll do well and you'll be surprised and pleased at the quality of her voice. I have only one suggestion: When she completes the first aria, ask her to do a second. Then, if you think well of her voice, ask her to take a lead role in a future opera."

Carlotta showed up on time the next afternoon. Still confident, still radiant. She mounted the stage and with a cue to the pianist she began to sing. Just as I began to feel she might falter, her voice grew stronger, in the low register as well as the high. I looked at Sieh's face. He showed no emotion one way or the other. She completed the number. He asked her to do another.

Carlotta was pleased.

At the conclusion of the second aria, Sieh went to her and in a soft voice said, "We will be in touch with you and soon." He was a man of few words. This was no "Don't call us, we'll call you" routine. Carlotta sensed that he wanted her to sing for him and she was overjoyed.

Several months went by. At last Sieh had a spot for her. She auditioned for a lead role in a great opera not often done in this country. He gave her the leading role. She received excellent reviews in the New York *Times, Opera News,* and an Italian-neighborhood paper. Her performance was a triumph.

Several weeks passed. At last, Carlotta came by the parish house, not simply to thank Mr. Sieh and me for what we had done for her, but to bid us good-by. She had received offers from several opera houses in Europe for the next season and had accepted. She was leaving for Italy within the week.

"It was a mistake to leave the career I had made for myself in Europe. But the bitter experience here has been good for me."

She shook hands with both of us. Laughingly and with joy in her voice, she said, "However, if I had not come back to the States, I would never have met either of you. . . . You make a good team. Someday, I hope we meet again."

As Carlotta left the office that day I handed her a leaflet which long ago I had printed to give to singers (and writers) with her problem. It is the familiar statement of Sergei Rachmaninoff, the world-famous pianist and composer. It is a description of Rachmaninoff's experience with a hypnotist, Dr. N. Dahl. Rachmaninoff was despondent, depressed, and unable to function, yet with Dr. Dahl's assistance he was able to produce the magnificent Concerto No. 2, Opus 18. Rachmaninoff wrote in his *Recollections* the following tribute to Dr. Dahl:

My relations had told Dr. Dahl that he must at all costs cure me of my apathetic condition and achieve such results that I would again begin to compose. Dahl had asked what manner of composition they desired and received the answer, "A concerto for pianoforte," for this I had promised to the people in London and had given it up in despair. Consequently I heard the same hypnotic formula repeated day after day while I lay half asleep in an armchair in Dahl's study. "You will begin to write your Concerto. You will work with great facility. The Concerto will be of excellent quality." Although it may sound incredible, this cure really helped me. Already at the beginning of the summer I began again to compose. The material grew in bulk, and new musical ideas began to stir within me—far more than I needed for my Concerto. By the autumn I had finished two movements of the Concerto—the Andante and the Finale. The two movements of the Concerto (Op. 18) I played during the same autumn and enjoyed gratifying success.

I felt that Dr. Dahl's treatment had strengthened my nervous system to a miraculous degree. Out of gratitude I dedicated my second Concerto to him.

6. The Minister—Fear of Dying

We had finished a great meal at one of New York's better seafood restaurants. I had noticed that Mac had been somewhat preoccupied during the meal. Contrary to his outgoing personality, he had been forcing conversation. Before the waitress brought the check, he leaned over the table and said in a strained voice, "I've decided to leave the ministry."

I laughed and said, "Take me with you."

My friend was the Rev. Dr. Macdonald Dodd, senior minister of one of New York's strongest and most influential churches. He was a man some ten years younger than myself; despite the age difference, our interest and commitment to the pressing needs of our churches, as well as those of the city, had brought us together in a genuine and lasting friendship. Before we left the restaurant, he convinced me of the sincerity of his intentions. I said, "Come around to the church tomorrow sometime before noon. I want to hear more of the details that led up to this decision and also what plans you have made for the future."

He agreed.

Unlike on most days, I was not crowded for time, and neither was Mac. We sat facing each other in comfortable chairs and I let him talk. The confession at first came slowly, then in a torrent of words.

"I have been in the active ministry twenty years and have faced just about every problem a parish minister can face: criticism of my sermons, criticism of my children, programs in education and worship that are empty and meaningless, members who use their 'Christian' influence to retain the status quo and to ignore the needs of disfranchised people, churches which become self-serving and which would rather retain the institution than be a servant of the people—all of this I have been able to absorb.

"However, thus far I have been able to live with many paradoxical situations because I have known that in leaving the church and taking another position, say on a college faculty, I would be confronted with similar if not identical problems. But I am leaving."

Mac was leading up to something; I was beginning to feel the suspense. What had he done? Another woman? Misused church funds? I knew he was one of the best preachers in New York, a popular-scholar type. He was liked and respected even though many of the positions he took on a variety of issues were contrary to the opinions of many members of his congregation. So I waited.

"Wes, for the past six or eight years, I have been sinking deeper and deeper into depression—the focal point of my despair is the inability to accept as fact my own death."

He told me the name of the psychiatrist he had seen for a while. He was grateful that the doctor had helped to some extent to pull him out of his depression, but when he returned to a more normal state the aspect of death appeared to him to be even more devastating.

I said, "You mean that you feel worse now about death and your own dying since the depression has somewhat lifted."

"Exactly so. I keep arguing with myself. 'Why am I overemphasizing death?' 'Why do I keep brooding about death?' 'Why am I possessed of this irrational fear of death?'"

Sitting before me was one of the strongest and ablest men I have ever known—a fellow minister who had since college and seminary days read, studied, and written about death, who every week went into hospitals and nursing homes to comfort the dying, who every week conducted at least one funeral service and who was compelled by the nature of his position to bring hope and counsel to the bereaved.

"How do you feel about your own death? . . . Can you contemplate it? Are you afraid to die?" Mac asked.

"Since I outgrew the fear of the dark as a child, I have had no fear of my own dying."

"I don't believe that."

"Why should I play games? Why should I lie to you or to myself? I despise old age with its grotesque distortions of the body and mind . . . but death, no."

Mac said somewhat sarcastically, "I suppose you're one of those who insist that a dying man can die bravely and triumphantly with a smile on the lips."

"That's nonsense," I said. "I came into this world by coercion and kicking and screaming—I probably will go out the same way. Jesus did not go out with a smile on his face. 'My God, my God, why have you forsaken me?' were several of his memorable words on the cross. . . . Joan of Arc, heroine of history, left screaming; Michael Servetus, Calvin's stain, a strong and noble Christian man who refused to accept the orthodox theory of the Trinity, cried and screamed while being burned to death at the stake."

"You just said that you were not afraid of death . . . yet . . ."

"It's not the last few weeks or the last hour in which I am interested. . . . Stalin, the butcher of millions, may well have died quietly in his sleep. What matters, Mac, is that for more than forty years I have had peace with death. When I think about it, I experience no perceptible feelings . . . certainly not of fear or dread."

"Do you believe in reincarnation?" Mac asked.

"At one time I thought I did. . . . Reincarnation has an explanation for genius. It has an explanation for those *déjà vu* feelings, the feeling that we've been in a certain place before. Reincarnation has a sensible interpretation of justice: we get it in the neck here if we've been bad in a previous life. If we suffered in the previous life, we have it easier in the present. We receive what we deserve, no more, no less."

"Sometimes reincarnation makes sense to me; at other times . . ."

I said, "If reincarnation has the correct interpretation of justice, then Jesus in his previous life was a selfish, brutal hellcat, the same for the Apostle Paul, the same for St. Francis of Assisi."

I then changed the subject. "How do you feel after conducting a funeral service?"

"Drained, devastated . . . and it's getting worse. The death of a young child or adult used to break me up. Now I feel the same about a funeral for anyone . . . he or she may have reached ninety. What am I going to do?"

"You asked me a question about my fear of dying and also whether or not I believe in reincarnation. . . . Let me ask you a question. 'Do you believe in God?'"

He said, "If I wanted to be argumentative, I would ask you to define 'believe' and 'God,' but I think I know what you mean."

"I hope you do. Both of us long ago gave up the belief in God the celestial bellhop, God the universal Santa Claus, God who is 'up there' or 'out here,' etc."

Mac said, "Having gone through the 'Death of God' phase, I came out with a stronger faith in God."

"That's good—two disciplines will assist you in overcoming the fear of death."

"Two?"

"Yes. One is theological, the second is practical. When you believe in God—not in the 'doctrine' of God, but in God—you accept the life cycle which He has set for all of life. That cycle concerns a beginning, a middle, and an ending. Once this seeps into the subconscious, there are many psychological implications as far as death is concerned. God, not man, thought up the idea of living, which includes dying. There is purpose in the cycle. Whatever God wills about death is more than acceptable to me. If He wants death for me to be the termination or obliteration of life, I accept that with no reluctance. If He wants me to continue in the next life where I leave off here, I accept that. If He has a heaven whose streets are paved with gold, I accept that. If He wants me to do a little time in hell, I accept that. . . . By the way, He also will be in hell. You know the words better than I: 'If I ascend to heaven, thou art there, if I make my bed in hell, thou art there.' Such a commitment has nothing to do with getting prepared for the last week or the last year—nothing to do with dying bravely, triumphantly, a smile on the face. It simply means that I have accepted God, the source of creation and the ground of all being. Whatever He wills, I want."

Mac was quiet and looked at me for a moment. "I have come a long way since my 'Death of God' days, but I have not come that far. . . . You said that there were practical aspects toward acceptance of one's death. What are—?"

"There are three. When you have done these, the natural acceptance of death is accomplished."

"What are they?"

"First, making out a detailed will; second, writing instructions concerning the type of funeral service you desire: church funeral service, church memorial service, funeral home, or private; third, writing a detailed request concerning the disposition of your body: *to science, burial* in the ground in a cosmetic casket, surrounded by a vault, or *cremation.* You have these options and you should make your preferences clear."

As I talked about these unthinkable things Mac's face turned white, he gripped his hands, started to speak, and then choked.

"Take it easy, Mac," I said.

"Get me a glass of water. . . . I'm sorry."

I hurried to the cooler and brought him the water. He was pacing the floor. "My God, my God," he kept repeating.

"I'm sorry if I upset you," I said.

"You not only upset me, but in talking about the will, my own funeral service, and the disposal of my own body, you ripped me apart."

"I shouldn't have done it."

"You touched sensitive nerves. God, I have made peace with. And all that theological jazz you were discussing . . . I can accept. But the thought of my body lying and rotting in a stinking casket six feet underground, or being cut up by impudent, fun-loving medical students, or being pushed into an oven and burned like an old rag— this really hit me."

He stopped pacing and sat in the chair and slowly finished the glass of water.

I said not a word. Silence between friends is sometimes the tie that binds.

At last he said, "Wes, there's one subject that our friendship has never permitted us to discuss."

I nodded and knew what he was about to say.

"This crazy hypnotic stuff you're mixed up with. I've always thought it was pure trash and wondered how a man of your capabilities could have been conned into it. . . . Now I don't know."

"Nearly all of my close friends, in and out of the ministry, hold with different degrees similar views concerning hypnosis."

"But there's something I did not tell you. . . . The psychiatrist who helped me with the depression stood me on my ear. He said as soon as I felt better, perhaps I should try hypnosis. That's what he said." Mac paused for several minutes. I remained silent. "I don't think I can be hypnotized, but if I can, do you think it could help me out of these sweats—these childlike fears?"

"They are not childlike . . . they are demonlike. Yes, I do believe the hypnotic process can deal with these fears. It may help when all else fails."

"When can we start?"

"We'll start as soon as you're ready. I want you to begin the hypnotic series at least with the vocabulary." I took a huge book from my shelf and said, "Read this carefully." The book was written by an author both of us knew and respected: *Psychology, Religion and Healing,* by Leslie D. Weatherhead. Dr. Weatherhead was the world-famous pastor of London's City Temple. Though he was known the world over as a scholar, a renowned pulpit artist, and a biblical authority, few of his followers knew of his ministry in hypnosis. In the book I gave to Mac, Dr. Weatherhead takes three chapters to describe the history, theory, induction procedures, and applications of hypnosis, using case histories out of his own ministry at City Temple. Mac did not know about the hypnotic ministry.

I laughed and said, "If I am in Weatherhead's company, I may not be so crazy after all."

The reason I did not want to rush into hypnosis with my friend is the solemn fact that the three practical responsibilities which I wanted him to assume can create deeper anxiety in a death-fearing person, especially if the fear had become irrational, as it had in Mac's case. However, being able to perform these tasks does have salutary effects. In other words, the detailed writing of one's will can create a sense of relief. The suggestions of the type of funeral one prefers not only relieves the family of burdensome obligations but also helps one to accept more realistically that there is to be an end. Especially helpful are specific suggestions indicating whether the service will be a church funeral service, a church memorial service, a service in a funeral home (God help us), a private service in his home, or no service at all. In addition to these carefully written instructions, he should be as specific as possible as to the time element of the service, favorite hymns, favorite Scripture and poetry, if any.

The third task is the most difficult for the fearful to perform—instructions concerning the disposal of one's own body. Robert E. Neale in *The Art of Dying* expresses the thought cogently when he says, "The first fear is about the fate of the body. The picture of a decaying, rotting body is not pleasant. So we try embalming, sturdy caskets, and even graves lined with metal."

The next week Mac came for his first hypnotic session. "Weatherhead's book was fascinating. Wonder how I missed it? . . . Do you have another book on hypnosis?"

"There are about two dozen on my shelf. Take this one. . . . Are you ready for a trial run with hypnosis?"

"I'm more than ready."

Suggestions of induction were simple, easy, and soothing: eyes closed, pleasant sense of heaviness so that the body will feel as if it were sinking into the couch, relaxation of various muscles of the body. He was soon ready for the first posthypnotic suggestion. I gave Mac some important homework. "This week you will go to your attorney, explain to him that you have never made out a will. You now desire to do so. When you have completed the details, you will experience a tremendous sense of relief. You will become almost euphoric."

I brought Mac out of the trance. He was a responsive subject, though there was some twisting and turning of the body during this first session. However, when he came to full consciousness, he immediately said, "I don't think I was hypnotized. . . . I heard everything you said; I could have opened my eyes at any time."

"That's what it's all about; you never lose complete control, and you hear distinctly what is being said. . . . Do you remember the posthypnotic suggestion I gave you?"

"Sure. . . . I'm to go to an attorney this week and make out a will. Furthermore"—he threw back his head and laughed, the first real laughter I had heard from him in months—"and in going to the attorney I'm supposed to feel great, euphoric."

"That's about it," I said. "Come back for your second session next week."

Mac left my office chuckling to himself. Hypnosis was working!

The next week we followed the same procedure, except that the homework was to bring in a detailed account of his own funeral. He responded beautifully, but once again said, "I can't believe I was hypnotized."

We were ready for the third session.

"Now for the last posthypnotic session. It matters little whether you remember this or not. The point is, you will carry out the instruction in a calm and cool manner, feeling nothing more than if you were writing a grocery list. Next week you will bring in a written, detailed account of the manner in which you want your body disposed of. The options are before you—traditional burial, body to medical science, or cremation."

He came out of the trance easily. We chatted about a ministers' luncheon we were to attend the next day. He left the office.

Next week he brought to me a detailed account of the disposal of his own body. I was curious to see which of the options he had chosen. It was to medical science, a beautifully written document. The body would not be used as a cadaver; rather, various parts would go to certain institutions and the remainder could be used by a medical school in any way which the authorities saw fit.

After I looked the paper over, I said, "Mac, I want you to read this aloud to me. It is beautifully done." Of course, I did not want to hear it read because it was "beautiful"; I wanted very much to study his face, his composure, his reaction to reading the description of the disposal of his own body.

"Sure thing," he said. He read the paper in a rich, mellow voice. I watched him closely. There was no twitching of the face, no jerkiness, no sign of fear.

I was satisfied that here was another example of how the amazing power of hypnosis can quietly but surely assist one who suffers from an irrational fear. When Mac completed the reading, he put the paper on the table next to the couch. He was silent for a moment, then his face broke into a big smile. He looked straight at me and said, "I still don't believe I was ever hypnotized. . . . It was our friendship that did it, and I want to thank you for giving so much of yourself when I desperately needed it."

People who believe that in the hypnotic process the autonomous self must be sacrificed will never accept the fact of hypnosis—no matter to what degree they have been helped.

II
Sexual Disturbances

1. The Masturbator and the Great Cover-up

I sat reading the Sunday paper, dozed a little, and halfheartedly watched a television program. The program was entitled "Sex and the New Woman." It was a panel talk show, a moderator and four women. The panelists were physicians and psychologists. I must admit that when the women warmed up to their subject, I tossed the paper aside and came fully awake.

There was a question from a high school-age girl in the audience and it was addressed to the four panelists. She first made a statement, then the question. "All of us have been relieved to learn that masturbation for both men and women is a good and necessary function. My question: Can masturbation be indulged in so frequently that either physical or psychological harm will result?"

Each panelist took a shot at answering this question for the young lady and for a nationwide audience. Each gave virtually the same answer. The psychologist said that she was delighted that we have arrived at this place in time when such a question could be raised in public. She further said that masturbation by both sexes has been going on a long time. There were no tests and no literature in our day which indicate that masturbation can be harmful. In fact, when indulged in on a regular basis, it is a lifesaver for the otherwise sexually deprived person. The other panelists agreed, and one of the physicians added a spicy bit of personal testimony. She said, "When my husband is away for any length of time, I masturbate once a day, sometimes twice."

As the program wound down, my thoughts turned to Gary, a man in his middle thirties whom I had been seeing in the office for several months. Gary, divorced for more than ten years, was a tall, thin, and nervous man. He had inherited a fortune from a distillery industry and had never worked a day in his life. He owned apartments in London, in Paris, on the Riviera, and of course in New York. After becoming better acquainted, he invited me to dinner at his Park Avenue penthouse. I accepted with pleasure. An elderly black woman prepared the meal and it tasted as if it were straight out of Antoine's of New Orleans. The woman came with his inheritance. In fact, she had reared him since early childhood, mainly in continental Europe. His parents were always traveling to distant parts of the world, so it fell to Aunt Ellie to care for him. He was an only child.

After dinner we went to the terrace, drank a glass of Drambuie, and resumed our discussion of his problem. Several years prior to his seeing me, he went to his family physician for an examination, at the conclusion of which Gary asked the doctor a question. "You say I'm in excellent health but I have a problem that I have never discussed with you. I masturbate once or twice, sometimes three times a day. My penis at its base has now developed a callus. It often becomes irritated. Am I overdoing the masturbation?"

The doctor, a man past sixty, threw back his head, laughed, and said, "I wish I had your problem."

He was stunned by the doctor's apparent indifference. He remained silent. The doctor noticed his discomfort and then said in a reassuring voice, "Seriously, Gary, masturbation is good for you . . . it's good for your health. If the penis becomes a little irritated, here's an ointment you may use." He handed him a small tube.

In my office the first time Gary was quiet, reserved, and almost noncommunicative. At last he opened up and told me the story of his masturbating habits. I asked him if he would resent several questions pertinent to the subject, and he said it would be all right. So I asked.

"How long have you masturbated on a daily basis?"

"More than twenty years . . . since I was a teen-ager."

"Does it interfere with your sex life with women?"

"Oh, no—no, not at all."

"See many women?"

"Two or three times a week."

"Intercourse that often?"

"Yes."

"No difficulties with erection, penetration, or ejaculation?"

"None."

"You want to slow down the masturbation and you believe hypnosis can help you."

"That's right . . . so right."

I felt his eagerness for the hypnotic session and said, "Tomorrow we'll give it a try."

He was on time the next day. Though nervous, he soon entered a medium trance level. When the time was right, I said, "Gary, open your eyes and look at me." This he did. "Blink your eyes when necessary and let's talk. We'll talk as easily as we did a few minutes ago. Understand?"

"I understand."

"Do you see many women?"

"Not very many."

"Have intercourse with any of them?"

His voice began to shake, but he answered, "Not often."

"What do you mean by 'not often'? How long has it been since you attempted intercourse with a woman?"

"I can't remember."

"A year?"

"Longer than that."

"Five years?"

"Just about."

"Do you have strong sexual fantasies?"

"Yes."

"Mind telling me about them?"

"I see naked men and women feeling me and playing with me."

"Then you masturbate."

"That's right."

I brought the session to a conclusion. "Close your eyes, lean your head against the pillow, and let go of all the tension."

He came several more times to my office. I was working on the theory that his compulsive masturbation was due mainly to being tied into knots. If hypnosis could relax him, slow him down and give him confidence, perhaps the masturbation would be retarded and he would in reality, not in fantasy, ease his problem. However, hypnosis did not work with this compulsive masturbator. I beg to differ with the lovely ladies on the TV panel show who talked so enthusiastically and noncritically about masturbation. "All you want" seemed to be their consensus. When masturbation becomes compulsive it produces a variety of ills, most of which are difficult to treat. It may also become a way of deliberately avoiding the real thing. It was about this time that Gary invited me to his penthouse for dinner.

As we sat on the terrace, I needed another Drambuie. What I had to say now would be a shocker. I wanted to say it sympathetically but firmly.

Within the past ten or fifteen years male and female homosexuals have gained a great deal of acceptance and freedom in our society. However, we should not delude ourselves; there are still unreasonable restrictions and community oppression in many places and in many forms, even in New York and California. Myths abide in great numbers: "Homosexual teachers will corrupt our children." We never stop to think how many heterosexual teachers take advantage of students on both high school and college level!

"Homosexuals are weak and cannot be trusted." From certain biblical characters to historical men and women in music, art, and science, from Oscar Wilde to novelist Merle Miller, homosexuals have demonstrated they are as strong, as gifted, and can be trusted as much as the rest of the population. "Homosexuals are sick." A moment of reflection may destroy this myth. Of course, some homosexuals are sick, but so are some heterosexuals. I marvel that the average homosexual does not show more instability than he does. If you, the heterosexual, woman or man, were forced to live the furtive, secretive life that most of these people of the other gender live, you, the heterosexual, would be an emotional wreck—afraid of losing your job, afraid of being kicked out of your apartment, afraid of losing close friends, afraid of going to church, afraid of parents who cannot and will not accept you as son or daughter.

I have known sick homosexuals, but the reader will surmise from reading this book that I have known and dealt with some very sick heterosexuals! Most homosexuals are not "gay"; they are sad people who are forced to live the furtive life, they know what it is to live in the closet.

The last myth is that homosexuals and Lesbians can be changed. With a dose of psychotherapy here, a little religion there, with time and patience, and perhaps a marriage, they can be changed. We must distinguish between the homosexual and the individual who from time to time engages in some form of homosexual activity. The latter may be strongly *heterosexual;* for example, if he happens to be in prison, he may find a sexual partner of his own gender. However, when he is released, he will immediately seek the company of the opposite sex. His stronger preference will assume its natural role. The former, on the other hand, he too having served time in prison, upon being released will also pursue his sexual preference . . . homo with homo, Lesbian with Lesbian. As these words are being written there appears to me to be an effort on the part of a variety of promoters to blur the image of sexuality, so that being bisexual, AC–DC, is the "in" thing. I have counseled dozens of male homosexuals and a number of Lesbians, I have listened to dozens upon dozens of sexual stories of both homosexuals and heterosexuals, and without exception the sex preference eventually reveals itself. Experimenting with bisexuality has been engaged in throughout history (Hirschfeld, Havelock Ellis, Kinsey, Masters and Johnson). However, authorities such as those just mentioned agree that "preferences will out." The American Psychiatric Association has recently given reinforcement to my long-held views: The genuine homosexual is not sick and he or she will not be changed. It is far better to get him out of the closet, help him to accept himself, and take the risk with a hostile society.

Gary said, "How do you like my view?"

"It's breathtaking," I said.

"Wonder why hypnosis did not work for me? Was I really a good subject?"

"You are an excellent subject."

"Then why?"

My answer had to hit home. This was a direct confrontation. No more cat-and-mouse, beating around the bush, no more games. "Gary, your problem is not masturbation, this is a cover-up. You are a closet homosexual."

He blanched, almost dropped his glass. "How do you know?"

"You recall our conversation when you were not under hypnosis?"

"Yes."

"Do you recall our conversation on the same subject when you were under hypnosis?"

"Yes."

"Did you realize you were giving me opposite answers to the same questions?"

"I remember . . . but for some reason it did not bother me."

"It was after the next session that I was sure your basic problem was not masturbation."

"I left my wife for this reason. I should have come to you years ago."

"Perhaps you're right."

"Could we have several more hypnotic sessions?"

As kindly as possible I said to Gary, "Your real problem is getting out of the closet . . . coming out in the open. This is a new day we're living in. You don't need to flaunt your sexuality; neither must you fear it nor be ashamed of it. Hypnosis is a worker of miracles, but your problem is one it cannot touch, much less cure."

"Where do I go from here?" he asked.

"I will see you in additional counseling sessions if and when you admit first to yourself that you are a homosexual. We can begin work from that point."

The moon was full, the lights over the city hung like multicolored constellations. Gary stood; I stood. His face was firm, his voice steady. He shook my hand and said, "I'm ready to begin as soon as you have the time."

I saw Gary for almost six months. He came out of his New York closet. He now lives in England most of the time . . . and he does not live alone, and he does not masturbate three times a day.

2. The Blast-off Comes Too Soon

Premature ejaculation is a form of impotency. The important question is: "When is ejaculation premature?" A young woman of little sexual experience went to her doctor and complained of her husband's deficiency in this regard. Since her husband was to see the doctor, she felt it only right that she have the opportunity to tell her version of their sex problem.

The doctor wasted little time. After a few preliminaries he put the following questions to her. She reconstructed them for me in this fashion:

"How often do you have intercourse?"

"Three, sometimes four times a week."

"Do you both enjoy foreplay?"

"Yes, very much."

"Approximately how much time in foreplay?"

"It varies . . . sometimes just a little, at other times as long as thirty or forty minutes."

"How many minutes after penetration does your husband ejaculate?" the doctor asked.

"Sometimes ten minutes, sometimes fifteen."

"If your husband can indulge in reasonable foreplay, can have intercourse three or four times a week, penetrate, and hold off ejaculation for ten or fifteen minutes, he is a sexually remarkable man."

I agree with the doctor.

Harold, at age forty, was into his third marriage and was having trouble. Real trouble. He was plagued with the worst form of premature ejaculation that I have ever known or read about. He could stand a minimum amount of foreplay, was easily excited, and had to ejaculate immediately. Ejaculation took place as the penis touched the outside of the vagina. His third wife of six months was disgusted. She would no longer use the pill, diaphragm, or any other form of contraception. Her attitude was: "What's the use? He comes before he gets it in."

Harold's wife insisted that he wear a condom, just in case. Pitifully, he said to me, "I often come now as I begin to put the condom on."

In most cases, this type of impotency, as opposed to non-erection or retarded ejaculation, yields itself to hypnotic suggestion with considerable ease. I was not so sure about Harold, his was a severe case. However, with poker face, I kept my doubts to myself.

Harold was a short, dumpy little fellow with a moon face. He worked as an accountant. His problem had plagued him since his early teens. Sometimes it was better, sometimes worse. He had been to a round of doctors and sexologists. One advised him, "Relax. You must relax." He said to me, "How in the hell am I going to relax? It's like hearing a dentist, who is burring a hole in your tooth near the nerve, say, 'Relax.'" Another advised him to masturbate five minutes before intercourse. Harold said this didn't work because when he ejaculated, it was over as far as he was concerned. A sexologist advised him to keep his mind off sex while he was undressing and especially as he approached his wife. He could think of the ball game his team won or lost, make up in his mind a long list of things he was supposed to do the next month. "This is screwy. How do you keep your mind off sex when she's naked in bed waiting for you?" Another bit of advice: "Let your wife assume the top position, you assume the passive role." Another: "Take two or three shots of scotch about thirty minutes prior to." The last suggestion brought a grin to Harold's chubby face. "With the scotch, I could not get an erection, so I fell asleep." Harold was not a drinking man.

So hypnosis for him was the place of last resort. Had I seen very many people with his problem? "Yes," I said. "Do you think you can help me?" I answered, "In all probability." He asked, "How many sessions will it take?" I said, "A minimum of six."

The first session did not go well. Harold was trying too hard. He was desperate. He wanted very much to be a good, responsive subject. I said to him as he was about to do the "breathing of sleep" exercise, "Do not strain. Take it easy. Do not attempt to follow everything I say. From here on, it doesn't matter whether you remember or not. Touching the subconscious will release within you powers you never dreamed you possessed."

By the time we reached the third session, Harold was a picture of relaxation. I made the suggestion that his hands were not only heavy but cold, very cold. His response to this was instantaneous. He was now ready for a strong posthypnotic suggestion.

"Are you right- or left-handed?" I asked.

"Right," he said in a soft voice.

"The suggestion I give you applies to both hands, especially the right. As you approach your wife tonight, you will notice that the right hand will become cool, cooler, and then cold, as cold as it is now. For the time being eliminate all foreplay. Ask your wife to stimulate herself manually. You do the same. You will notice that the coldness in the hand will be transmitted to the penis and you may have to work to get an erection. . . . Do not fear. The erection is a sure thing." I paused for a moment. "Harold, do you understand?"

"Yes."

"The next suggestion concerns the penis once you have penetrated." I then took from my pocket a quarter-inch rubber band. "Extend your right hand," I said. "Now your forefinger. Identify the forefinger with your own penis." I slipped the tight rubber band on the forefinger, all the way to the base. Circulation was almost suspended. With his cold right hand and extended forefinger Harold began to feel the stricture.

"You feel the tightness at the base of the forefinger?"

"Yes."

"You must visualize the forefinger as the penis."

"Okay."

"Immediately upon penetration tonight, you will experience a strange sensation. The penis will be cool, but at the base you will feel this severe tightness. So long as you feel the tightness, it will be impossible for you to ejaculate . . . impossible for you to ejaculate until you say, 'Come.' When you say, 'Come,' the tightness will disappear and you will experience your first ejaculation within your wife's vagina." I immediately slipped the rubber band off his forefinger. The finger had turned slightly blue. I then said, "Within one minute the temperature in your hand will return to normal; the tightness in your forefinger will be relieved. These will remain normal until you approach your wife tonight."

The next day Harold called me with great excitement. "I got it in, I really did. . . . I held it about three minutes, but the tightness at the base of the penis left me and I had to come."

"I think we're making progress. See you Friday."

At the Friday session the same procedure was followed. Suggestion of coldness in the hand, and the rubber band was made a little tighter. The same suggestion concerning holding and letting go was given.

Harold did not call me the next day. I was concerned that perhaps the procedure would not work for him as it had for so many others.

He kept his Friday appointment.

"Why didn't you call?" I asked.

"I wanted to surprise you with the good news. Each time we did it, I got stronger. Over the weekend, there was no coldness in my hand, no tightness at the base of the penis. I put it in, we remained still for a minute or so, slowly we began moving, then faster . . . within a reasonable time I let it come. . . . I let it come."

He reflected a bit and said, "That cold-hand suggestion and the rubber band on the finger really worked. I knew you were putting a rubber band on my finger." He laughed.

I said, "Harold, it wasn't the cold hand and it wasn't the rubber band. These were simply exercises which enabled you to gain *confidence* in yourself. The good old subconscious went to work for you and you discovered a *confidence* that you never dreamed you had."

Hastily he asked, "Do you think it will last?"

"If it had been only the cold hand and the rubber band, I would have my doubts, but since your capability is now rooted in *your* confidence, I can say with some certainty: it will last."

Harold, at age forty, was a bridegroom with a third wife. I have a hunch this marriage will last for quite a while.

3. The Impotent Husband and the Frigid Wife

Most of the time when there is marital trouble and help is sought by one of the partners, it is the wife who takes the initiative. However, in this case it was Oscar (everybody who knew him called him

Os) who made an appointment. He was in the brokerage business and that particular area of the financial sector was having its problems. When he came to see me, I thought his problem might be due to worry and anxiety about his declining financial condition. "No," he said, "I've enough put away to see us through this crisis, even if it lasts a year or two. It's my wife. She is so damned frigid that I just can't make it and it's driving me nuts."

Jo, his wife, was slightly younger than Os, who at the time was pressing forty-five. When the children went off to college, she took a position with the bank where she formerly had worked. She was of average weight and height, average good-looking, average attractive personality. She appeared to be a good-humored, easygoing woman. I had known both Jo and Os for about ten years.

"It's like this: every time I get ready, which now is about once every two weeks, she comes down with a headache, the familiar back trouble, or she's just plain tired from working at the bank. She won't even make an effort any more."

"That could be painful to the marriage." I said this because I could at the time think of nothing better to say.

"Wes, you know I'm not the kind of a guy that goes around with any available skirt. . . . I'm just not. Besides, I think a lot of Jo. In fact, I still love her after twenty-one years."

"Not surprised to hear that. . . . I always thought you had a superior relationship."

"But I reached the point . . . where I just can't get it up and I keep thinking maybe I could make it with somebody else. What do you think I ought to do?"

"There are several Masters and Johnson type of sex clinics in the city, perhaps you could go to one of them."

"I've thought of that. . . . Called two but they said both partners must come for diagnosis and treatment. Jo would not agree to go. You know Jo respects you. Would you agree to see her?"

"She may like me, but this is a sensitive area. Do you think she would come to my office?"

"I'll talk to her tonight and call you tomorrow."

"Os," I said, "if you call me, it's no good. . . . If she calls, that signifies that at least she senses there is a problem and wants to do something about it."

"I believe she'll call you."

The next morning Jo called. We chatted about their two children now in college and about her going back to work. She was delighted to get out of the house and into the world . . . made her feel alive again. At last she said, "Os told me he had been to see you. . . . I would like an appointment at your convenience."

We set the time—five o'clock Monday of the following week. Jo came looking less dowdy, less "average," and more attractive than I had seen her. She wasted no time in getting to the point. "Wes, we've a real problem. Just two years ago, about the time Os's business went bad and I went back to work, he appeared threatened. He never was a demanding sex partner—in fact, most of the time his performance in bed was poor even when we were younger. But then it happened. One night when both of us appeared in good spirits, no liquor or anything, just good spirits . . . we got into bed, reasonable amount of foreplay, and then, as was our usual position, I lifted myself on a pillow, he made the effort to enter . . . as he did so, his face turned white, his penis went absolutely limp. I reached down with my right hand and squeezed it, hoping that he could achieve sufficient erection to get it in . . . but it was impossible.

"He jumped off the bed and with a snarl said, 'Goddamn you, you've made me impotent.'"

She paused for a moment.

I asked, "Had he ever had this experience before?"

"As I indicated, he never was what I would call great . . . getting an erection was somewhat difficult most of the time . . . but my little maneuver of squeezing three or four times enabled him to get an erection sufficient for him to ejaculate and me to reach orgasm."

"What has been the pattern since that night when both of you were feeling good but he was unable to make it?"

"We tried about two weeks later. This time he got an erection, penetrated, went soft in thirty seconds."

"How did he react?"

"It was the only time I thought he was about to strike me. But he didn't. He just got up, dressed, got in the car, and drove around for about an hour."

"That's it?"

"That's it . . . for nearly two years. I admit I've never been too eager for sex, but, my God, I never thought I would sleep in bed celibate with the man I love for a period of two years. . . . I'm beginning to feel it."

"Had you ever shown signs of frigidity?"

She thought for a moment. "Yes, there were times when I felt no desire for sex, and he approached me with amour, and I guess I turned him off."

"You forced yourself, without enthusiasm, without orgasm?"

"Of course, I faked it . . . as hundreds of other women do."

"Did he ever know?"

"Only on two or three occasions. I was a poor actress. . . . He knew."

"Could both of you come to my office at the same time?"

"Yes, but not simply to talk about our sex lives! Since we were married we've read every sex manual published . . . this position, that position, feel her here, kiss him there . . . we need a hell of a lot more than mechanics and technique."

"A few of the newer sex books stress more than technique," I said.

"I simply don't believe we can be helped by more reading or more instruction or more talking. . . . We need something that will enable us to capture the spark, something to move us."

"You're probably right."

"For a number of years I've been reading about hypnosis. Some of the accomplishments are indeed beyond explanation."

I was not prepared for Jo's cooperation, much less her enthusiasm about hypnosis. "We ought to set an appointment as quickly as possible."

"That's easier said than done. Os does not believe in hypnosis. He puts it in the same class as the occult . . . talking to the dead, fortunetelling, etc."

"I never knew he felt that way about hypnosis."

"He thinks you are a great counselor and he feels we need good counseling, which at this stage of the game is horseshit . . . excuse me, please, Wes. . . . I didn't mean to offend."

I hid a smile. "No offense."

"We need something to give us the incentive, the motivation, the confidence, the desire."

"You've spelled it out word for word."

"I'll talk to Os tonight and call you in the morning. I'll call you if he's willing to come for hypnosis."

"If he's not cooperative, I must refuse to see either of you. *He must make the call for an appointment.* If he does, I'll be glad to work with you together."

"I think I can get him to call. . . . If anything can help two sexual cripples, I believe it is hypnosis," said Jo.

For a number of years I have counseled married couples having serious problems. It is wicked to oversimplify any problem, and I certainly do not intend to do so with Jo and Os. However, having seen the deterioration of so many marriages, I keep chasing the reasons why this is so. Do people now live together so long that the prospect of a fifty-year marriage seems frightening? Is it money? Is it the difference of opinion as to how money is spent and who will have veto power? Is it the perennial in-law problem? Is it children or the lack thereof? Is it sex, with one enthusiastic and the other indifferent? I am sure that all of these factors have something to do with the near dissolution of the family as we know it in the Western world. However—and here I am about to oversimplify—couples who know how to use language, who know how to verbalize, who know how to communicate thoughts, feelings, and fantasies, have a built-in weapon against marriage disposal. I know couples, married thirty, forty, and fifty years, who by some miracle share this remarkable trait of talking to each other. A cynical friend of mine says that in any restaurant he can tell the married couples from singles simply by the way they talk or don't talk to each other. Maybe so. However, verbal communication may not be so easy as I have indicated. For one thing, it must have the spark of spontaneity. If one of the partners is inclined to filibuster each time they get together, this is sure death. If the circle of conversation is forever on such items as clothes, cars, jewelry, the end is in sight. If one partner is poorly informed on all subjects and the other is well informed on many subjects, this too is an inhibition. If one partner is obsessed with only *one* subject (say, investments in real estate, gold, bonds, or certificates) and the other is equally obsessed with only *one* subject (say, religion or children), alienation is just around the corner. If one partner is compulsive about "my" analyst and the other could not give a damn, marriage stability becomes shaky.

So I make a simple observation: When two people in a marriage or in a meaningful relationship spontaneously have something to say to each other, staying together becomes easier than parting. Within a few years a man may forget those one-night "lays" when he was on the road. He is likely not to forget that charming woman with whom he talked till two in the morning.

Jo and Os, married twenty-one years, ran out of gas. Early in their marriage they began to force conversation, then they gave up. Certain symptoms preceded frigidity in Jo and impotence in Os. Their inability to talk to each other applied to sex as much as or more than it did to any other area of their shared lives. They could never discuss the subject to any extent except for Jo saying, "I'm menstruating," or Os saying, "I'm beat, exhausted." There was no intimacy or appreciation of the miracle of each other's body, no indication of preference for a position or positions, or practice of the ramifications of oral sex, and most serious of all, there was no sharing with each other their fantasies about sex. For years sex to Jo and Os was to get in bed about once a week or once every two weeks; a few minutes of "foreplay," then he would penetrate (when possible), she would reach orgasm (when possible), and that was that.

When Os called to say he was willing to come in and discuss their problem and that he was more than willing to go for hypnosis, we made the appointment. They came in a few days later and we immediately got to the business of the hour. Sometimes it is more difficult for a counselor to discuss intimate problems with friends than it is with total strangers. However, it was not so in this case. Jo was carefully dressed and looked comfortable and self-assured. Os would not have looked well dressed no matter what he wore; he was somewhat ill at ease, but ready for a hypnotic session.

As we moved into the conversation, Jo laughed and said, "I guess we're just too old for kid stuff. All of my friends my age are 'in the same boat.'"

Os commented, "I think we have a problem and I'm not ready yet to give up on sex."

"That's because you have the twenty-year itch," she said.

I interjected at this point something about communication as outlined above.

Os said, "You've hit the nail on the head as far as we're concerned. No communication on any level except bills and the children."

"I've often thought how good it would be to be married to a man where we could talk with enthusiasm instead of retreating into our own monastery or instead of flying into a rage at each other over a difference of opinion."

"Your comment, Jo—'how good it would be to be married to a man who . . .'—leads me to the core of our conversation. There will be no hypnotic session today. Instead I want you to do some homework. I hope it will not be embarrassing. . . . It should be fun."

Both now listened intently.

"Between now and Tuesday, our next session, go to the typewriter and put on paper your innermost thoughts on the subject: 'How good it would be to be married to . . .' This will include customs, habits, communication, and above all fantasies, especially your current sexual fantasies. Write what you feel; make it as pornographic as you like."

Os said, "I don't believe I could do that. . . . Suppose somebody other than yourself saw the paper."

I said, "Anonymity will be observed. In referring to other people in your paper, only initials are to be used. You will sign the paper in code. Os will be 'O' and Jo will be 'J,' the paper will not be dated, nor will it be addressed to me. . . . Each of you will bring your own paper to me Monday. I shall study them and from them determine whether I believe hypnosis will be helpful in your case."

Jo exclaimed, "I think the idea is super. Just great. I'll write a book between now and Monday."

As they left, I shook hands with both of them but said to Os, who

I sensed would have greater difficulty, "Put it all down; get it all out."

Monday, the papers were in. I was surprised. Os had done much the better job, neat, well organized, and an amazing amount of honest description. Jo's was good, but written too fast, and I felt she was hedging at certain points, except when she came to fantasies.

Both papers, in the beginning, covered virtually the same material . . . early marriage, long years of drudgery, the coming of the two children, Os's success with his business, their friends' struggles in marriage, separations, divorces. When it came to sex, they were explicit; fantasies were revealed in detail.

Os made the point of how much he loved Jo, how he envisioned her in so many different ways. . . . In bed they would take their time, he would become erect and she would play. In fantasy her body became to him a fascinating miracle; the descriptions of positions were erotic and stimulating. Os desired more than any other thing to have Jo take him orally. On and on he went with his desires and fantasies.

Jo's paper skipped most of the early problems in their marriage. She described one experience when she almost went to bed with B.J., one of their close friends. Then she came to her sexual fantasies, and of course they included Os. In even more detail she contradicted her blasé statements about being over the hill, sex being kid stuff. She laid it out. "I see him coming to me, he fondles me, touches every part of my body. Then his hand begins to rub my ass, then with swift strokes he begins to pepper my soft skin until a slight pain is experienced. He turns me over—the kisses now reach every part of my body, my neck, my ears, my breasts, slowly his tongue goes down to the valley of my belly until at last it reaches that place of all places, that small exciting organ which explodes time after time—I do not want him to stop—I reach and reach and reach. . . . I say, 'Now, darling, it's time, put it in. . . . He puts it in, holds for a minute, we both abandon ourselves in wild thrusts until, wrapped in each other's arms, we lose consciousness as simultaneously we come together. We're still, he slowly withdraws, moves to his side, tenderly takes me in his arms, and says, 'Jo, I love you very much,' and I whisper, 'I love you with all my heart.' "

This is a summary of each paper. When they came in Tuesday, I congratulated them on their frankness. "Both of you have active fantasies. . . . That's good."

"Where do we go from here?" Jo asked.

"Neither of you know what the other has written?"

"That's right," they said in unison.

"I shall give the papers back to you—but with your permission, Jo will read and study Os's and vice versa. . . . Is that agreeable?"

Os hesitated for a moment.

Jo said, "That's okay by me. I think we should know how the other feels. . . . God knows we haven't been able to talk about it during these twenty-one years."

Os then said with a degree of enthusiasm, "Sure, I think it a good thing to see what the other said. Will there be any hypnotism today?"

"No," I said. "If all goes well, hypnosis will take place the next time we are together. Take the papers home, read them tonight. . . . No matter how aroused you become, do not attempt intercourse. Touch and rub every part of the body except the privates —kiss, French-kiss if you want—but remember no penetration, even if Os gets an erection. . . . It will not be his last; he's just beginning."

They wanted to come the next day; my schedule made an evening appointment necessary. As they entered the office and sat on the couch, each of them smiled and said together, "Wow!"

They had no idea that each felt as described in the papers.

"It was revealing, wasn't it?"

"I'm going to put Os's in my secret scrapbook."

"What happened last night?" I asked.

Os said, "We nearly drove each other crazy. . . . After reading each other's paper, we stripped quickly and made love."

"Did you get an erection?"

"I had an erection before I finished reading Jo's paper."

"Did you penetrate or have an ejaculation?"

"No," said Os, "but I could have any minute, but you said to hold it, and I did."

Jo looked at me quizzically. "I must confess after reading Os's paper I was uncontrollable. He sucked my breasts and I enjoyed two enormous orgasms. For the first time in my life I let *him* and all *my neighbors* know it!"

"Os," I said, "you've the makings of the world's greatest lover. . . . I think you're ready for a hypnotic session."

Two people are as easy to hypnotize as one. They followed induction suggestions—eyes closed, five deep breaths, heaviness of hands, the "breathing of sleep." They were excellent hypnotic subjects. Now for the application. I have tried the following posthypnotic suggestions with couples many times; only in rare instances have they failed. It went like this: "Tonight when you go home, take your time, shower, talk to each other. . . . You certainly have questions and comments concerning our counseling session and your papers, but talk about anything, get the verbal communication going. When you retire, Jo will remove Os's clothing piece by piece, Os will remove Jo's clothing piece by piece. . . . Understand?"

They nodded as they went deeper into the trance.

"Get in bed, no nightclothes of any kind. With these suggestions, you will easily fall asleep. . . . Both of you are still in the hypnotic state, completely relaxed. . . . You will remain in this relaxed state throughout the night. . . . Do not touch, do not make love. Lie naked together. Just before sleep say in a loving way, 'Good night, Os'; 'Good night, Jo.' Are you following me?

"Now for the goodies. Both of you indicated that you not only fantasize a reasonable amount but you have an active dream life . . . that's all to the good. You will dream tonight vividly, as vividly as if the acts were literally taking place. You may not remember what I now suggest . . . that, too, is all to the good. Your dreams will center around the material in each other's papers. If extraneous material comes in, that's also all right. The main thing is that the basic points in the papers will prompt the dreams and your subconscious will take over from there. Tomorrow night for the first time in almost two years you will be ready for your experience of satisfying penetration, intercourse."

I slowly brought them out of the trance. "Take your time, your mind will be bright and clear, your body will remain beautifully relaxed."

I said, "Jo, do you remember most of what I said?"

Jo: "Everything until we reached the breathing of sleep. . . . I faintly remember something about dreaming . . . but no details."

Os: "I stayed with you until you said something about taking off our clothes. I don't recall anything past that."

"That's great. Go home, chat with each other . . . you will sleep better tonight than you have ever slept."

They left the office happy to the point of euphoria.

My phone rang at seven-thirty the next morning. "Wes, this is Os. Rather not talk to you on the phone. . . . Can we come by your office on our way to work?"

A sleepy voice said, "I'll see you at eight-thirty."

I met them at the office; my secretary had not yet arrived.

Os: "My God . . . what dreams I had. . . . I awakened this morning about six with a tremendous erection. . . . I looked at Jo, she was awake, waiting. She said, 'I never had such a wonderful night's sleep. Are you ready?' 'Yes,' I said."

Jo: "All I can say is . . . it was wonderful. Never again will I put sex down!"

I laughed and said, "Two things: don't be gluttons, and don't forget to verbalize."

They left the office holding hands as if they were teen-agers.

4. The Rape Victim—She Had to Know

Vickie was graduating from college in June, two months away. I would miss her because she had been my best typist. During her four years with me I had written a variety of manuscripts on a number of subjects. Not only was she a speed artist at the typewriter but she was accurate, and even more important, she could decipher my peculiar form of using dots, dashes, arrows, "go back two pages," "go forward three pages," "skip this sentence and put it in the first paragraph," etc., etc. I would miss her.

She was small and thin, wore horn-rimmed glasses, and in recent years had been harassed by a stubborn form of acne. She had already accepted a teaching position in a little village not far from her home town. As far as I could tell, she had few friends—boy friends or girl friends. She was somewhat shy, an excellent student, and the first person in her family who had graduated from college. She would make a good teacher, and in spite of her shyness, I felt children would love her.

One day late in April she came by my office. I was busy with boring matters, and it was good to hear her say, "Hope you're not busy. Just wanted to stop by and say hello."

My reply: "Come in, you've saved me from the worst tedium of the ministry." I was going over budgets and wondering how we would make ends meet the rest of the year. So it was a relief to see Vickie and to chat with her about graduation and schoolteaching instead of checking typing material.

We went into my private counseling room, and when I had shut the door she said, even before sitting, "I've been wanting to talk with you privately for the past two years . . . but I don't have much courage."

"I'm glad you made it. Say on, Vickie." The smallness of her body and especially the tiny face made her appear fifteen instead of twenty-two.

"If you have the time, I'll get it out—it has taken me a long time to come here like this. . . . I'll do it if it kills me."

"It won't kill you."

She then told me the following story. I listened with no questions and no interruptions.

"Two years ago this spring, I was walking from the dorm, down the hill to the gym. We were playing an important game that night. It was about 7 P.M., and the sun had not set.

"One of the fellows, who I am sure was a senior, approached me and we began an easy conversation. 'We gotta win this one,' he said. I was surprised at how naturally I said, 'We sure do. . . . This game determines whether we go to the championship playoffs, doesn't it?'

" 'It does. . . . What's your name? Mine is Jim Poppular.'

" 'Mine is Vickie Smith.'

" 'Most of my friends are trapped in the frat house . . . suspended from all social activities for a week—too much booze. Let's sit together.'

" 'Okay by me.' It was a relief to have someone I could go to a game with . . . especially someone I could talk to. Besides, in the growing shadows, I could see that he was tall and probably hand-some.

"We arrived at the gym, spoke to several students, and found seats on the top tier. Our team won.

"After the game was over, he said, 'Let's go over to the Hut and get a hamburger.'

"Without a second thought I said, 'Sure.' I had a final paper in biology to complete over the weekend, but that was no sweat.

"We walked away from the gym and toward the Hut. Instead of going the longer way, which had been recently paved and lighted, he suggested we go the short way on a small path that led through high grass and overgrown bushes of various sorts. Know the place?"

I nodded.

"The entire area from back of the gym to the street, about two city blocks long, is secluded. Necking, petting, etc., take place with considerable privacy. The moon was barely to be seen, the April night was unusually warm, and I was feeling safe and accepted. About midway to the street where the foliage was deepest, Jim took my hand and squeezed it. I squeezed his hand back. Then we stood still, he reached down, drew me to him, and kissed me. I did not kiss him back, but said, 'It's short notice for that, isn't it?'

"Dr. Shrader, you have reason, I suppose, to believe that my sex life and my relations with men have been nil . . . and you would be almost correct. However, I'm not a virgin. I had two brief en-counters in high school and three here as a freshman. I cooperated each time, but the experiences left me feeling like a nothing person. I had the idea then, and still have it, that I would never have sex with any man I did not intensely care for. I may not be frigid or sexless, but the whole business means far less to me than to most people. I've had no sex in three years, and I must say I have not missed it."

She took off her owlish horn-rimmed glasses. The acne had almost cleared up, and she was positively attractive. As is some-times the case, Vickie, short and thin, possessed oversized breasts. In all the years I had known her I never thought of her as physically attractive. She had a delightful smile and a quick, intelligent mind.

She was speaking in a controlled voice as if she were describing how she planned to put together the biology paper.

"I barely got the words out—'It's short notice for that, isn't it?'—when Jim grabbed my arm, twisted it in back of me, and in a lowered but gruff voice said, 'Don't yell or I'll break your arm.'

"I was stunned. He pushed me off the path into the brush. I started to yell, and he said, 'Goddamn it, I mean it. . . . It may not be your arm but your neck.'

"I remember vividly everything I had on—jeans, blouse, light sweater, loafers, panties and bra, no stockings.

" 'We're going to do this as if you were cooperating all the way. . . . Take your clothes off, beginning with the sweater, blouse, and bra.' I said nothing, but hesitated. At that point he thought I would refuse. Out came a knife—I heard it click and then felt it at my throat. Huskily he said, 'If you do not do as I say, you've had it.'

"I removed my sweater, blouse, and bra. His hands touched my breasts. He repeated, 'My God . . . oh my God, what . . .' Then he pulled me to the ground and began sucking the breasts, first one, then the other—still keeping the knife at my throat. I was frightened beyond control . . . and became nauseous. Within minutes he pulled off my jeans and underpants. He mounted, I heard him panting louder and louder; I felt pain as his penis penetrated. I cannot remember how long it was before he ejaculated—it must have been a very short time. He continued to lie on top of me, the knife at my throat. I had not screamed or uttered a word. 'Now he will kill me,' I said to myself. But he didn't.

"Within two or three minutes, he whispered, 'Take this handkerchief, clean yourself up as much as possible . . . put your clothes on, and keep your mouth shut.'

"I did as directed. After I dressed, he carefully brushed grass and thistles from my clothes. 'Comb your hair,' he said. With his left hand he handed me a comb. . . . The knife was still held in his right hand near my face. By this time I was numb but had the feeling that maybe he was not going to kill me. He said, 'I'll walk you to the street. We separate there . . . go straight to your room . . . if you tell anyone about this, including your roommate, the knife will be waiting.'

"He was not lying. There was a split moment in the bushes when I was slow in opening my legs and I felt the knife . . . he almost hit the vein then. Now I was convinced that if I reported the act or talked about it to anyone, he would never be satisfied until I was dead.

"We came to the lighted street, and I got a good look at him. He went one way, I went in the opposite direction, four short blocks to my dorm. Dazed and still frightened, I went to my room . . . straight for the sink. I vomited my insides out. Then I threw myself on the bed and re-created the entire scene. . . . He seemed more out of his mind as he sucked my breasts than when he penetrated. That's just about all."

I spoke for the first time. "Vickie, after two years, why have you told me this story?"

"I already feel better, just getting it out to someone. . . . Hope you don't mind. You're not disappointed in me, are you?"

"On the contrary, my admiration for you knows no bounds. It would have been terribly unwise for you to act in any other way than that which you have described."

Not once in the telling of this blood-curdling story did she lose her composure or stumble for words or break down. Vickie was a remarkable young woman.

"There's still more to the story," she said.

I nodded and said, "Take your time."

"The man told me his name was Jim Poppular. . . . There was no senior by that name and there was no one in the student body by that name."

"I guessed that. . . . You could have gone to the Registrar's Office and asked permission to look over the pictures of the entire student body. . . . You would not have to tell the office the real reason for so doing." The college was quite small. It would have been easy to pick his picture out of the files or even from the college yearbooks. The senior book for the year was already out. However, it was possible that the man was not a student, or he could have been a dropout who had returned to see the important basketball game.

"How could I pick out his picture?"

"Why not?" I asked.

"For the reason that from the moment we reached the street that night and I was free of him, my memory of what he looked like vanished. Even though we sat side by side in the gym for two hours, I have no recollection of the color of his hair, the contours of his face . . . big mouth, little mouth, big nose, little nose. I cannot even remember the kind of clothes he was wearing."

I said, "That would have made it embarrassing if you had decided to report the act to the authorities . . . not being able to furnish *one* detail of his physical features except that he was tall."

Hurriedly, she said, "No one could have dragged me to the authorities. . . . Even if I had become pregnant, I would have had an abortion and kept the matter to myself. As far as the man who raped me is concerned, he is safe from being exposed by me . . . for a variety of reasons, one of them being that my mind blanked out. I've no recollection of him whatsoever."

Vickie had typed two or three of my papers on the subject of hypnosis. I knew what she was leading up to. "Do you think under hypnosis you could help me see the man's face? I want to know who he is. . . . I really do."

"Why not let the matter drop? You seem to have handled it well during these two years. Recall may simply make you more unhappy."

"If you think I cannot handle the situation, you're mistaken. More than anything in the world I want to see that man's face again."

She left the office, waved good-by, and said, "See you Friday."

Forcible rape is one of the most brutalizing experiences any woman ever endures. By forcible rape I mean the act of intercourse without consent. A woman may not struggle and fight—the perpetrator may be holding a six-inch knife at the jugular vein—she may lie still with not a whimper and without attempting to scratch the violator's eyes. She may have had sexual contact with dozens of men prior to the rape; she may or may not have gone to a doctor or reported the event to anyone, even her best friend. It is forcible rape when the act has taken place without the victim's desire or consent. When by threats, intimidation, or physical violence, the act occurs—this is rape.

What stupid myths and jokes has the male perpetuated concerning this act. "God Almighty, you should see the way she responded once I got it in." "She kept hugging and kissing me." "She asked me when we could do it again." "You should have seen her when I tore her panties off and when I took out my Big John—she was hot and eager." "And, man, when she started to come, you could hear her squeal a block away."

Is the rapist insane? Some are and some are not. Is the rapist sick? Some are and some are not. I am convinced that though many cases of rape are committed by men who are sick, the act is committed every day by men who are as normal as most of us. Why does such a man do it? It is not because he is being sexually deprived—not in our day! Is it to prove his masculinity? Is it out of a feeling of rage at women, all women, but most of all that one woman who gave him birth but denied him love? Is it simply to have one more thing to boast about—an ego trip?

For whatever reason, there is no experience that leaves a woman more devastated. The results are often horrendous. Some women despise sex from that moment on. Some women, even though they have not been torn or ripped, continue for years to experience pain in the vaginal area though there is clinically no reason for the pain. Some become totally frigid. Hidden fears turn off all sex valves, so that even when she finds herself with a reasonably considerate man whom she likes, it is impossible for her to have an orgasm. Some may have an orgasm, but not if her beloved penetrates—he must remain outside. Some women throw an armor around their emotional lives. They become suspicious, hard, insulated from the world.

Is it any wonder that a woman, young or old, hesitates to bring charges? From her hospital bed or in the police precinct house, she must tell in detail what happened. If the rapist is located, she must identify him and tell the story again to her lawyer; on the witness stand she must again go through the nightmare . . . for judge, jury, attorneys, witnesses. The chance of *proving* that she was raped is indeed small, less than 5 per cent. The state of New York has recently passed a law which may be helpful in this respect; namely, a law which abolished all requirements for corroboration of the victim's testimony. The fear that many men will be trapped by women who claim that they were raped, when actually they consented, would be ludicrous if it were not tragic. The difficulty is that a woman who has been raped cannot bear the glare of publicity and a court trial. She would rather keep the bloody mess to herself than go through legal procedures. It remains to be seen how many women will be running down to court claiming falsely to have been raped now that they do not have to produce witnesses! My calculated guess is that the increase will be minuscule.

One other deterrent measure has been adopted by New York as well as other states. This is setting up special rape patrols consisting of women only. The first contact with anyone immediately after the act is the most difficult. In those communities which have female rape patrols, the first recounting of the story can now be told to a woman, a woman who understands in a way that no man can understand.

Vickie was back in my office two days later for her first hypnotic session.

"You have no fear? No hesitation about hypnosis and what we may uncover?"

"None. . . . I trust you . . . you are more than a father figure: I see you as my real father who has been dead for eight years. Please believe me."

"I believe you." From the articles which she typed for me, she was thoroughly familiar with my procedures. However, I explained to her that after induction the process of regression was the application we would follow.

"I'm ready when you are," she said.

"All right, get yourself comfortable. Eyes closed and take five deep breaths."

I made several suggestions about the hands becoming heavy, the eyelids extremely heavy. Into the "breathing of sleep" she went. Here the suggestions of being at peace, of becoming drowsy and sleepy, take effect. With no fear, Vickie moved into the most responsive category. The subconscious was taking over.

Then I said, "Vickie, as you go back the past two years, we'll first dwell only on those things at college which have been pleasant and which you have enjoyed the most.

"When I ask you a question, you will answer it in a clear, strong voice. Speaking will deepen the state of relaxation rather than weaken it. Beginning with September of this year, your senior year, tell me the three most enjoyable experiences you have had."

She replied clearly, "That's easy. One has been working with you. I have learned so much that I would otherwise have missed. Two, the field trips we took in connection with archeology. They were great. Everybody in the class liked what they were doing, and Professor Gregory is tops as a teacher. Three, my work with the children in student teaching. . . . I have been teaching the fourth grade and have enjoyed every moment of it."

"During your senior year have you enjoyed going to varsity games, such as basketball?"

She frowned slightly. "I have not been to a basketball game or any other type of athletic game for two years."

"What about friends? Made any lasting friends, men or women?"

"No . . . not even my roommate. We keep our distance. It's better that way. You asked about friends. . . . I have made a few friends at the school where I am teaching . . . members of the faculty and mothers."

"That's wonderful," I said. "Now let's go back to the beginning of your junior year."

She interrupted me. "Oh, yes . . . I was crazy about all sports, I wanted very much to make friends on campus . . . girl friends, but especially boy friends. . . . I've never had a close boy friend, a relationship. . . . Understand?"

"I understand.

"You're in an excellent frame of mind. Let's go directly to the basketball game, the last one you attended."

Her body twitched slightly, but she said, "I'm ready."

"You walked to the gym with someone you thought was a student, a senior."

"That's right."

"You reached the gym. What then?"

"We stopped and chatted with several students and then climbed to the top tier . . . good seats."

"Was your roommate at the game?"

"No, she went home for the weekend; mother died."

"Vickie, there's no point in reviewing the unpleasant scene in back of the gym. I want you—"

"I agree."

"I simply want you to tell me about the scene at the gym. . . . Make no effort at using your memory. Just let it happen. Reconstruct the events: the gym, the players, the crowd. Did you know anyone sitting near you?"

"Sure, several students."

"Can you give me their names?"

"Bob Granger and Sally Brown . . . just in front. . . . Down about two rows were Irving Schwartz, Bruce Kemple, Buzz Biagaloni, and Marge Piper."

"Can you see them clearly?"

"As if it were today."

"On what side of you was the student, the senior, sitting?"

"My left."

"Again I say . . . let it happen . . . do not strain the memory. We will simply unlock the trapdoor and memories which have been buried will come forth. Can you see him clearly now?"

"Yes, very clearly."

"How was he dressed?"

"In corduroys, tan; turtleneck shirt that matched."

"Tell me about his physical features."

"He was tall, his face was long and very masculine . . . fair complexion; hair was beautiful, light red. He was cleanly shaven, very neat. He laughed easily, even with his eyes . . . the bluest eyes I've ever seen."

"Had you ever seen that man before the night of the basketball game?"

"Of course."

I could hardly control the excitement I felt. However, when you've done hypnotic work as long as I have, you learn control, and you know enough not to be surprised.

"Where?"

"He's Amy's—my roommate's—fiancé. . . . They are to be married at graduation."

"Tell me his name."

Without faltering a second, she said, "Tom DeWitt."

"Do you have any idea why you told me his name was Jim Poppular?"

"None . . . none at all. . . . Wait a minute . . . wait just a minute. . . . Jim Poppular was the name of the high-school student who first introduced me to sex. I hated him. Why did I identify Tom with him?"

"You were suffering from a form of hysteria. When this occurs the mind does strange things. For Jim Poppular's sake, it is just as well that you never told anyone about the incident."

"You are *so* right." She was getting tired. Her head moved downward and her voice was somewhat softer.

"Rest for a while, lean back, keep your eyes closed, and bring to your mind pleasant scenes and pleasant thoughts."

She rested in peace; everything was soft, easy, comfortable, safe and secure.

"When I count to five you may open your eyes. . . . Your mind will clear up, you will recall our conversation in detail, every bit of it. Your body will remain relaxed."

I counted to five. She opened her eyes, was quiet for a few moments, and then said harshly, "I'll be damned . . . Tom DeWitt. How could I have blanked him out so completely? . . . The whole scene in the gym and behind the gym is now clear. Why am I not jumping and screaming?"

"Your level of acceptance is extremely high. . . . So, Tom DeWitt . . . president of the senior class, captain of the soccer team . . . good student," I said.

"You knew Tom, did you?"

"Yes," I said, "I remember him. For a variety of good reasons, several members of the faculty and I suspected that it was he who, in his junior year, violated one of our freshmen girls, but there was no proof."

Vickie said with bitterness in her voice, "I wonder where the bastard is now."

I said slowly, "Tom went into the service immediately after graduation. I don't think he and Amy ever married."

"So he's in the service."

"Yes, he was killed in Vietnam six months ago," I said.

"It couldn't have happened to a more deserving guy."

Vickie, the girl who never lost her composure, reserved and untouchable, made this statement in as cold and vicious a tone as I have ever heard. She had thrown about her emotions an impenetrable armor. The deed of two years ago was past but still alive. Never again would she allow anyone, male or female, to reach her except for superficial, meaningless friendships.

5. The Rape Victim—She Could Not Forget

Angie lit another cigarette, crossed her legs, and said, "I cannot get the son of a bitch's face out of my mind."

During the year she had remarried and happily so to an official in the city government. She developed no sexual hang-ups from her ordeal and aside from smoking too much—which she insisted she would never give up—seemed to be in excellent emotional condition. Angie was an author and our friendship dated back to a chance encounter at the annual meeting of the Author's League four years previously. Her new novel had just been accepted, so she was in a good mood. However, she was harassed by the image in her mind of the face of the man who raped her one month before she was married.

"Why did you go to his apartment?" I asked.

"He has a home in Cleveland Heights, Ohio, and an apartment here, East Sixties. We were introduced in the office of —— Publishers. He indicated that I might just be the person he was looking for, someone who would write a piece of dialogue for him . . . said dialogue was to appear in a national magazine. For this I would be amply compensated. Since I was two-thirds toward completion of the novel, and since I was to be married within four or five weeks, and since I needed the money, I jumped at the chance to be associated with him on the project.

" 'Meet me at my apartment at two, Wednesday afternoon. We'll outline your assignment.' He gave me his address."

It is not uncommon in New York for women to go to an apartment of an analyst, psychiatrist, podiatrist, osteopath, etc., who employs no secretary, nor may there be anyone in the apartment except the professional and his client. So Angie did not give the matter a second thought. She accepted his invitation and was in his elegant apartment at two, Wednesday afternoon.

I said, "I think I know the name of the man. . . . Cal Karpen?"

"Yes. How did you know?"

"I have followed him on speaking trips to a number of campuses where his primary contribution was to rape one or more women students."

Angie continued, "I know his track record now—I did not know it then. . . . Well anyway, when I arrived at the apartment, he greeted me cordially, offered me something to drink. I took a cup of coffee and then we got down to the business of the day, or so I thought it was the business of the day. He explained the outline and synopsis of the work he had done. 'I'm rotten at writing dialogue. . . . All you do is ghost about three thousand words.' We agreed on a price, more generous than I expected. I drank another cup of coffee and we chatted amiably for several minutes.

"As we talked I began to feel uncomfortable in Mr. Karpen's presence. He was short, powerful, and looked younger than he was. His head was too big for his shoulders and he constantly gesticulated. If he said, 'It's a nice day,' up would go his right hand and arm. . . . As you probably know, his left arm has been amputated. As with the gesticulation, when there was nothing to gesticulate about, so it was with his nervous, sarcastic laugh."

"If you were uncomfortable, why didn't you get up and leave?"

"This I did; I gathered my papers and indicated that I had another afternoon appointment. It was early fall, my coat was in a hall closet just across from a bedroom. He preceded me to the closet to get the coat, laughing nervously all the time. As we reached the closet, he suddenly pushed me into the convenient bedroom.

" 'You're not going quite yet,' he said in a commanding voice.

"I was frightened but managed to say, 'What in the hell do you think you're doing?' He locked the bedroom door and put the key in his pocket.

"I saw immediately the position I was in: I was no virgin, but neither was I a tramp. I was thirty-nine years of age, and a divorcée. I had accepted an invitation to his apartment in the afternoon. I now knew he would attempt to rape me, but the thought went through my mind, what would I do afterward? Would there be a jury in the country that would convict a man under such circumstances? I even doubt that I could have secured the services of a reputable lawyer! A *News* headline would probably read: DIVORCÉE CHARGES CAL KARPEN WITH RAPE, and in lowercase type: *In His Apartment*. Then would follow in detail the ridiculous story of my being raped by a one-armed man in his apartment at two in the afternoon. By the way, his right arm was powerful and had strength beyond that of the average man. With that arm he shoved me a third of the way across the room and onto the bed.

" 'Take your underclothes off—and your shoes. . . . Kneel, facing the side of the bed.'

"As my body landed on the bed, thought patterns swifter than light crossed my mind—my options were before me. He appeared not to have a weapon—I could go for his eyes, kick at his testicles, scratch his face. . . . If I attempted any of these he surely would strike back—a battle would ensue. The thought of my marriage just a month away now flashed before me. That settled it. When he snarled, 'Hand me your shoes . . . take off your underclothes,' I did as he directed. He said, 'Kneel on the floor . . . face this side of the bed.' He quickly removed his pants and shorts and sat on the bed, I kneeling between his legs. I still thought of striking him, of making a bloody battle of it, but something stopped me. . . . I caved in.

"He demanded oral sex. 'You've got more to lose than I have. . . . I know about your marriage, I know you have been with other men, including Dan Bossy, who used to work for me.' Then the abominable, sarcastic laughter. He got his oral sex, such as it was—he was impotent! Within two or three minutes he demanded that I lie on the bed. He tried to get it in, and I suppose he did, but it was partially soft, a slight erection, no ejaculation."

" 'That's enough,' he said, and pushed himself off me. 'Get dressed. Go tell your friends, go tell the police, go tell your boy friend that Cal Karpen raped you in his apartment.' "

Angie continued, "Of course, during this entire year I've told no one about the incident. I'm not a child, I have fought men before, I know the Upper East Side scene, but none so psychotic as this."

I said, "You want my help. . . . I assume it is for something more than telling me this tragic-pitiful story."

"You've helped several of my friends in a variety of ways. Can you get the picture of that man's face out of my mind?"

"I've done it before. . . . I see no reason why I would fail with you."

"When do we begin?"

"Wednesday at two." I grinned. Angie laughed at the words "Wednesday at two."

Of all the worlds I live in, I find authors and writers to be the best-informed persons on a variety of subjects. An author who writes about plant life will likely be an informed man on a number of subjects; the same is true for one who writes mystery novels. It so happens that I live in the world of the church, the world of music (opera), the world of the theater, the academic world, the world of travel, the world of psychotherapy and the world of writing. Angie was a good writer. She had read and written a great deal about mind control (which she considered a con game) and biofeedback (which she admired). She was a well-informed person on many subjects, but now she, the writer, found herself emotionally trapped.

Previously I indicated *induction,* putting a person in a hypnotic trance, is relatively easy; almost anyone can do it if he has confidence in himself and is working with a cooperative subject. However, it's the application of hypnosis that matters—WHAT IS DONE AFTER THE SUBJECT IS HYPNOTIZED. Angie knew about induction but was unaware of the process involved in removing the face of lust from her mind; however, she was more than ready for any suggestion I made.

The method I chose was one that depended on conditioning and reconditioning the subject. I saw Angie six times and each time we followed the same process until at last the face was gone, never to appear again.

Angie was a responsive subject; easily and quickly she reached a deep hypnotic level. It was a simple task to help her reach the point of hallucination, which means the object is either changed or appears not to exist. Karpen was a nationally known figure. His pic-

ture was in the paper that very morning. I cut it out; the picture
would be useful working with Angie.

When she reached what I considered her most relaxed state, I
said, "Angie, in just a minute you will open your eyes. . . . Instead of the trance being broken, it will be deepened. Now open
your eyes and blink them when necessary." She did as instructed. I
held the picture in my hand, not more than two feet from her face.
"You recognize this man?"

She recoiled and said, "Yes, it's Karpen."

"Take it easy . . . you will lose all tension and anxiety . . . you
will be able to look at the picture without feeling anything."

She nodded.

"I'm still holding the picture and you're still staring at it. . . .
Watch carefully—slowly, gradually the picture will become the face
of a clock. . . . Beginning now, Karpen's picture fades and the
picture of a clock appears . . . slowly, slowly, slowly. What do you
see now?"

The process of hallucination was beginning.

"Face of a clock."

"Does the face have hands?"

"No, just the face of a clock . . . numbers but no hands."

"Watch closely. . . . The short hand begins to appear, it points
toward two, gradually but surely, it appears. . . . Do you see the
hand?"

"Yes."

"Now another hand begins to appear. . . . It's the long hand of
the clock, slowly, slowly, slowly . . . now. The long hand points toward twelve. . . . Do you now see both hands?"

"Yes, very clearly."

"At what time are the hands of the clock set?"

"Two o'clock."

"No longer the face of a man . . . the face has faded . . . in
place of the man's face you now see the face of a clock, set at two
o'clock. . . . Angie, can you hear me clearly?"

She nodded.

"Whenever and for whatever reason the face of Cal Karpen
flashes before you, *in that instant the face of the clock will appear*.
The hands are set for two o'clock. This will be a reminder to you of

the pleasant hypnotic session you've had in this room. You will immediately experience a sense of relief and relaxation. Do you understand?"

"I understand," she said.

I brought her out of the trance, asked her to rest for a moment. Then I said to her, "Close your eyes and tell me if you can see Karpen's face."

She closed her eyes. . . . It was minutes before she replied, "Faintly, only faintly."

Angie came to the office at two o'clock each Wednesday for six weeks. Hypnotic conditioning completed our task by the fifth session. A final session was held to reinforce and assure her that the lecherous face of the man would never haunt her again.

III

Addictions—Three of a Kind

1. The Alcoholic—Water into Wine

Alcoholics Anonymous, as far as I know, has more success in aiding the alcoholic to find sobriety than all the physicians, psychiatrists, psychoanalysts, ministers, and counselors put together. When Bob called for an appointment to see me, I agreed. In true alcoholic fashion, he lied to me about the reason for his coming. He had a bad case of "nerves" and wanted me to calm him. At the second session he told me the extent of his problem, the seriousness of which I had been unaware of. He had been an alcoholic ten years, and was formerly the manager of a large supermarket. Now forty-four, he had reached low bottom. He was a night drinker, and the pattern was to consume a minimum of three quarts of wine between seven and twelve each night. He was a real "wino." When he began sneaking drinks before noon, the jig was up. His wife left him two years prior to my seeing him. His two sons, one in the service and the other working at a gas station, refused to have anything to do with him. He was now headed for oblivion.

When he completed his story, I said to Bob, "Let's get to an AA group as quickly as possible."

He was sober that morning and could muster a faint smile. "Off and on I have been in AA for five years. My longest period of sobriety was two months. AA is for many people but not for me."

Bob's problem of acute alcoholism is serious beyond description. Brain cells have been damaged, the liver eroded, and malnutrition, with a variety of side effects, has set in.

In telling about Bob it is necessary to give a detailed account of the method of induction I use with such difficult cases. This also includes the two other subjects in this chapter, the cigarette addict and the compulsive eater. Each of these three has an out-of-control problem rooted in severe compulsions which in themselves are often substitutes which mask deeper neurotic trends. Previously, I have said that it is the application of hypnosis—what the operator decides to do *after* induction—which is of great importance; however, in saying this, I do not mean to belittle the manner in which the hypnotic state is achieved. There are times when the operator can be too quick with a subject, or too authoritarian or too passive, too loud or too abrasive. A subject may be brought into hypnosis when such is the case, but the chances are his depth of relaxation and loss of tension will not be great.

The induction procedures described here in working with Bob, the alcoholic, are identical to those used with Gino, a four-pack-a-day smoker, and with Maria, the gorgeous but obese woman. The procedures I decided upon *after* induction in these three cases varied and each will be described. However, for the present, I want to detail the *induction* process with the alcoholic, the chain smoker, and the "stuffer." This process is somewhat lengthier than usual. There is a variation in the cadence of the voice; there is also a change in voice volume.

The subject does not lie down. This can be a threatening position to a person who is just being introduced to hypnosis. He sits comfortably in a chair or on a couch, feet not crossed but slightly separated, hands falling loosely on his thighs.

Bob assumed this position with eyes closed. The induction went like this:

All right, Bob, keep your eyes closed, and begin by taking five nice deep breaths. Hold the fifth one for a second, and come down with me as I count five, four, three, two, one. Let the last breath out slowly, and at the same time let your shoulders sag and your body become as limp as possible. Within about two minutes you will notice the beginning of a pleasant sensation as if you were easily sinking into the couch . . . sinking, sinking, sinking [slowly]. Your entire body will become heavier, beginning with the head. By all means be comfortable. If you want to move your head to the right or to the left, or perhaps permit the chin to move toward the chest, that's okay . . . it's comfort and ease we're after. Now turn your thoughts toward the right hand, which is lying loosely on your right thigh. Imagine a weight being put on your hand. You must feel the weight and see it. Think "heavy" with me; the hand is getting heavier and heavier [repeated several times]. Now turn your thoughts toward the left hand [same procedure repeated]. As we have talked about the hands becoming heavier, you will notice that your head is heavier. As your eyelids remain closed, let them become as heavy as they want to become. If it becomes a strain to open them, let them remain closed and heavy.

In order to become a real person, one who is in control of all his faculties, you must achieve three important objectives. The *first* is body relaxation. Already I see muscles in your face beginning to relax [suggestions of relaxation are given to various areas of the body, including throat, shoulders, stomach, thighs, and calves]. *Second,* you must achieve the release of tension. You will feel emotional energy oozing out of your body—sometimes pushing its way through the pores of the skin, sometimes out the extremities of fingers and/or toes. These extremities will have a tingling sensation. ["Tingle, tingle, tingle" is repeated in a monotonous tone several times.] The *third* objective is related to the other two but probably is more important. The anxiety level must be lowered. Within the mind, gaze now at a huge thermometer, graded from one to one hundred. When the anxiety level is extremely high, alcoholics become non-functioning, non-producing people. They cannot do their work, do not relate well with friends, sexual intimacy is virtually impossible. When the anxiety level is brought down to a manageable level, then they function, produce, relate. They begin to know relief and joy. Bob, you see the thermometer, your level is about eighty-five degrees. As I give the suggestion "down," watch the red mercury gradually descend. All right, *down, down, down* [repeated eight or ten times].

Up to this point you have succeeded to a degree in achieving muscular relaxation, reducing hypertension, and lowering the anxiety level. Now, one minute or more of deeper-than-normal breathing. This is the breathing of sleep—rhythmic and slightly heavier than normal. See yourself lying on the bed, you are dropping into deep, restorative sleep. Try to capture that pleasant feeling of drowsiness. Keep breathing—you are becoming *drowsy, drowsy, drowsier; sleepy, sleepy,* and *sleepier.* [This is repeated several times, the voice becoming softer until a whisper has been reached.]

Now breathe normally. This is the moment when the miracle of the hypnotic process takes place—that part of the mind called the subconscious emerges to take precedence over bodily functions, the five senses, and the conscious part of the mind. The subconscious is the dynamo of the personality. When used negatively, it is so powerful that it can trigger the emotions and bore a hole in your stomach; used constructively and creatively, it can bring *initiative and incentive* to a listless life, *confidence* in yourself as a human being, and *motivation* toward great and good goals.

To demonstrate how powerful the subconscious is, I want you now to enjoy a pleasant experience. Your body begins to feel warm; the warmth moves from the outside to penetrate the body, you will notice within less than one minute that the hands are warmer and warmer. ["Hands . . . warmer" repeated several times. With the back of my hand, I usually touch the subject's hand.] Your hands and body temperature will return to normal temperature within a few minutes. This is the power of the subconscious, and there is no end to its possibilities for good. Rest for a moment.

With this procedure, the subject is at a level of hypnosis where he will respond to constructive posthypnotic suggestions. I promised to say something about what is done *after* induction has been reached. Here is where the years of research, practice, and training prove invaluable. What type of suggestions should I give? Shall I resort to the aversion method? After all, I was dealing with a hardcore drunk, a real alcoholic. Aversion procedure is negative and sometimes is powerful. The suggestion is given that any form of alcoholic beverage will make the subject nauseated to the point of vomiting. The odor will be that of strong urine. If the subject attempts to take one swig, he will be sickened by the taste of urine.

When I was much younger, I often used the aversion method. But I found it to be counterproductive, even though changes in the five senses are easily produced by hypnosis. With the alcoholic we are dealing not merely with someone who is drinking too much liquor, but also with a sick person with strong neurotic trends. Within a short time he will usually break through the suggestion and begin drinking more than ever. So I have virtually discarded aversion, not only with alcoholics but also with cigarette addicts and others. With Bob (and many others) I resorted to pleasant, positive suggestions. The one I used with him was turning a glass of New York tap water into his favorite French wine.

The suggestion went like this:

Bob, I am holding in my hand a glass of tap water. Take it in your hand, hold it for several seconds, imagine yourself in your favorite restaurant. Before you lift the glass to your lips, put it under your nose, swill it around slowly. Gradually the distinctive smell of your favorite wine fills your nostrils. Keep teasing yourself with this odor for a minute or more, or until you cannot resist taking a good-sized drink. When you drink the contents of the glass, you will know that you enjoyed your favorite wine. [As Bob swirled the liquid under his nose, a pleasant smile crossed his lips. Within one minute he put the glass to his lips and swallowed. He was convinced that he was drinking wine, not water.]

We have just about concluded this session. Tomorrow you will move even deeper into a state of relaxation; the wine will taste better than it did today. Keep your eyes closed until I reach the count of five. You may then open your eyes. Your mind will be bright and clear, your body will remain relaxed, and you will be freed from all anxiety.

I saw Bob every day for seven days. The second week it was every other day. The technique of induction became shorter, but the water into wine was the method we stuck with. The first two days there was an unexpected reaction. He awoke each morning with a hangover! The hangover left after the two-day period. There was a minimum of withdrawal pains. Bob came to see me on his own. He wanted to be rid of alcohol—forever. He believed he could be helped through the power of hypnosis. As of this writing, he has achieved eighteen months of total sobriety. Though his family is still alienated from him, this disappointment has not thrown him. He recently met a widow his own age and they, together, appear to be making it.

2. The Trumpet Player—Four Packs a Day

Gino was a noted trumpet player; he was also a four-pack-a-day cigarette addict. He came for five hypnotic sessions over a period of five weeks. From the first session he has not smoked one cigarette— four packs a day, a chain smoker, and not one cigarette since the first session!

The brief incident I now relate took place as a happy and confident Gino was leaving my office after his fifth session. As I opened the outer door for him to leave, a well-dressed, short-haired, clean-shaven young man pushed his way into the lobby. I waved good-by to Gino and then the young man asked, "Are you the minister of this church?"

I said, "Yes."

He said, "I want to have a conference with you."

I said, "That will not be easy because my next appointment is in ten minutes."

He said, "What I have to say will not take longer than ten minutes."

"Righto," I said, "ten minutes." I took him into the office. He sat facing me. His face was stern and I felt his anger.

He asked, "Do you believe in the Bible?"

"Oh, yes," I said. "I believe in the Bible."

Again: "Do you believe the Bible is literally the word of God?"

"I believe the Bible contains the word of God. . . . If you are asking me if I believe that snakes and jackasses carry on conversations with human beings, my answer is 'No.'"

"Then you don't believe the literal word of God."

"Have it your way," I said.

"Do you believe in being born again?"

"Yes, I believe in being born again. . . . I was just reborn by the experience of the young man you saw leaving the building."

"But do you believe in being born by the Holy Spirit?"

"We would have to define our terms and that would take up more than ten minutes."

He was becoming angrier. "Are you saved?"

"Yes," I said. "I'm saved."

"Have you been saved by the blood of Jesus Christ which was shed on Calvary's cross?"

"If you mean, 'Have I been saved by the manner in which Jesus died, so utterly committed to his calling, his principles, his values, his sense of brotherhood and the abundance of love'—the answer is 'Yes.' "

The stranger rose from the couch. His mouth set, his teeth clenched. "Are you a hypnotist?"

He had seen on the bulletin board in the parish-house lobby the announcement: "Hypnosis Counseling Service."

"Yes," I replied. "I use hypnosis in connection with my counseling work."

Then his voice rose in a trembling crescendo. "You're not a Christian, you have never been born again, and you do not believe in the blood of the lamb. . . ." His face grew red as he shouted, "Hypnotism is the work of Satan. . . . If you are hypnotizing people, *you are not working for God,* you are a servant of Satan and doing his work!"

By this time I also had risen and confronted the stranger; I spoke to him face to face, my voice firm with conviction. "You and I would agree on many things concerning religion; the areas of disagreement you would make all-important, and I would consider them incidental."

"My ten minutes are up—I'll be going."

"Just one moment," I said. He started to leave. I reached out, grasped his arm tightly, and swung his body around so that he was facing me.

He demanded, "Let go of my arm."

"I'll do that in one minute. . . . Your ignorance of religion is exceeded by your total ignorance of the nature and function of the hypnotic process. When any deed of kindness is used to bring health—physical and spiritual—to one of God's creatures, that deed is of God and it is good. In this room, an alcoholic was restored to sanity by hypnosis, a minister afraid of dying was helped to accept his own death, the young man who just left here was on the verge of emphysema, smoking four packs of cigarettes a day. By the power of hypnosis he has not had one cigarette in five weeks. . . . You have your gods mixed up. This is not the work of Satan but of God."

I let his arm drop, he moved toward the door. I stuck out my hand, smiled, and said, "Shake, we're brothers."

Seething with anger, he refused my hand and stalked out of the building.

In New York, I contend with this type of confrontation, with variations, at least once a week.

Gino, the trumpet player, in his late thirties, was at the end of his rope. Three months before coming to see me, he had a thorough physical checkup. His doctor was impatient with him and rightly so. The last time he had been checked, the doctor said, "No more cigarettes . . . not one pack a day, or one half a pack, not even one. They must go. Your lungs are on the verge of a very serious condition." Once Gino quit for three days and another time for four days. Then, in a moment of tension, he reached for just one drag. He was soon up to four packs a day. The symptoms of the average cigarette smoker are quite noticeable. It is not as if one had a tumor which begins as small as a pinhead and gradually grows to larger proportions, sometimes with pain and sometimes without pain. Almost from the beginning, smoker symptoms begin to develop . . . irritated sinuses and irritated membranes in the nostrils, foul taste in the mouth, mushy gums, soreness in the throat; time goes by, then a hacking dry cough, then a wet cough with phlegm, then shortness of breath, so that he who was a great trumpet player becomes a hack; a great swimmer becomes a tired swimmer within a short distance; he who played championship tennis is now lucky if he can get through two sets. The lungs are covered with tar, then strange sharp pains occur in various parts of the body, usually beginning with the left arm. By this time the smoker is in serious difficulty. Tar and other substances have attacked his breathing apparatus; nicotine, innocent-looking in its colorless state, has attacked his veins, constricting them strongly, so that life-sustaining blood cannot flow normally throughout the body—this produces not simply shooting pains but often a blood clot, a stroke, or a heart attack.

Congress, after considerable debate and opposition from a powerful lobby, voted that the following statement must appear on every package of cigarettes: *Warning: The Surgeon General has determined that cigarette smoking is dangerous to your health.* This may be the understatement of all time. Cigarettes are dangerous, but they are also deadly in that they contain substances which slowly and subtly go about their business of damaging and destroying the human body. A young man of twenty-one once said to me, "What the hell . . . what does it really matter if I die at seventy-two rather than seventy-four? Cigarettes give me so much enjoyment that I will gladly sacrifice two of my most decrepit years."

Ah, but it's not just the last two years which are in the balances, it happens to be the last twenty, in some cases the last thirty. . . . To watch a strong, healthy friend wheeze and gasp for breath that will not come, to see a dear one sleep in a sitting position for years, unable to lie down because normal breath is impossible, to witness the results of a hemorrhage, a stroke, a heart attack from which victims may recover but never again to be real people . . . to see and smell fingers that have been stained a harsh brown, to see teeth and gums pulled and cut away, to smell a foul breath which emits its odor not only from the mouth but from the lower regions of the lungs. . . . If it were only those last two years of a withered life, perhaps one could settle for that, but that's not the way it is.

Gino knew all of the above by heart. He also knew that his trumpet-playing days were over; the little white demons had reached him in a disastrous way even sooner than he expected. "What am I gonna do? All I know is music."

I asked, "Did the doctor say either of your lungs had perforated?"

"They're covered with tar but no puncture . . . yet; he's concerned about the pains." He pointed to several places, including the left arm. "I guess I'm washed up. I got a peach of a wife and three kids . . . and I can't quit the damn things." Gino had kept his sense of humor and told me the following story. He caught a cab to my office; when it stopped for a red light, he noticed the driver scratching, itching, twitching his head as if he had a tic. Gino said from the back seat, "Fellow . . . what's the matter, you sick?"

The cabbie turned slightly and yelled back, "I quit smoking cigs and it's drivin' me nuts."

"How long you been off?"

The cabbie yelled again, "Five hours."

Gino shut up. He could not tell the cabbie that he was on his way to a hypnotist to talk about his own smoking problem. He did, however, put out the cigarette hanging from his own lips!

The induction process used with Gino was similar to that used with Bob, the alcoholic. He was a medium responsive subject, good enough to accept posthypnotic suggestions. In a previous *counseling* session with Gino, he had asked, "Can cigarettes interfere with my sex life?" Angela, his affectionate wife, had sexual desires far more often than he could satisfy them. There were times when he was unable to get an erection.

To this I replied, "As far as I know, no exhaustive study has been made of the effect of cigarette smoking on sexual capabilities. However, in the *Reader's Digest,* January 1975, there is an article entitled 'Is Your Sex Life Going Up in Smoke?' It is an article by Genell J. Subak-Sharpe, condensed from *Today's Health,* published by the American Medical Association. I suggest you get a copy of the *Digest* and read the article."

I took a reprint of the article off the table and read to Gino two short paragraphs:

> Joel Fort, M.D., Director of San Francisco's Center for Solving Special Social and Health Problems, which helps people both to overcome the cigarette habit and to deal with sexual maladjustments, automatically counsels smokers who complain of impotence to enroll in the center's stop-smoking clinic. The overwhelming majority of men who do so, says Dr. Fort, report their sex lives markedly improved. He gives the same advice to women who complain of lack of interest in sex.
>
> Dr. Fort theorizes that smoking impairs sexual performance in two primary ways: the carbon-monoxide intake reduces the

blood-oxygen level and impairs hormone production; the nicotine intake constricts the blood vessels, the swelling of which is the central mechanism of sexual excitement and erection. Dr. Fort also cites secondary effects of heavy smoking: lung capacity is reduced, cutting back on stamina and the ability to "last" during intercourse.

Gino said, after hearing these words, "I'll be damned . . . I was beginning to think I was over the hill. . . . Cigarettes may destroy my lungs, but by God, they're not going to take sex away from me!"

He was now hypnotically relaxed, the subconscious emerged, and he was ready for a strong posthypnotic suggestion which was based upon our conversation in the previous counseling session. "Gino, you will discover today the ease with which cigarette addiction can be broken. . . . You will leave this room a free man, no longer enslaved by the poison which has drained your body. To your incentive, the power of the subconscious will be added; to your desire to quit smoking, the power of the subconscious will be added; to your will, the power of the subconscious will be added; to your motivation to quit forever, the power of the subconscious will be added. You are not doing this by yourself . . . there is a strength beyond you . . . you feel it, you experience it. In addition to the help you receive, the compulsive urge to smoke will first diminish and then disappear. Hear me now. Every time you experience a strong urge for a cigarette, you will think of Angela, whom you adore, you will see her naked, waiting for you. . . . When the urge for a cigarette strikes you, this urge and energy will immediately go to that part of the brain which controls sexual stimulation. . . . *Each urge for a cigarette will result in an erection.* Do you understand?"

He said, "I understand."

I brought him out of the trance. He was silent for a long time. Then he laughed and said, "What do I do with an erection when I am on a gig and away from my wife?"

In good humor, I said, "That's your problem and I know hundreds of men who wish they had it. . . . Seriously, if you and your wife are together, take care of it; if you are on a gig [musicians' term for a job], you have means of self-employment . . . you can take care of that easier than emphysema."

At the fifth hypnotic session, just prior to my conversation with the handsome stranger who believes that I have not been born again, Gino said, without a trace of a wheeze or cough, "I'm not only off cigarettes, but Angela and I are having a wonderful time."

I walked him to the front door, waved good-by, and let the stranger in.

Gino has been unhooked; he can once again blow the trumpet with the best of them, and he and his wife enjoy a marvelous relationship.

Only rarely have I used the technique of application which I have just described in Gino's unique case. This was purely improvisational on my part and was dictated by the fact that Gino was becoming a non-functioning person. He was afflicted with two major problems, not one: cigarette addiction and sexual impotence. In resorting to this method I attempted to resolve two problems with one posthypnotic suggestion.

With most people suffering from cigarette addiction, I use the material outlined on the previous page omitting the suggestion concerning sexual arousal and adding two other suggestions. These are presented in the following manner: "I now give you two posthypnotic suggestions. It is not necessary that you remember what I shall say. You will do them compulsively. First, you will be aware of every small and every great reward you receive from becoming an ex-cigarette addict. For example, a small reward is losing your own offensive odor of stale tobacco. This will be accomplished within less than one week. Great rewards include the disappearance of throat irritation, and the hacking cough, and easier breathing. These usually occur within a period of three or four non-smoking weeks. It is not enough that you receive these rewards, you must be aware and grateful for them.

"Second, if you ever again reach for a cigarette, you will be highly conscious of what you are doing. It is quite possible that 50 per cent of all cigarette smoking is done unconsciously: after the meal, with a cup of coffee, at the telephone or typewriter and so forth. You will be conscious of touching the cigarette; you may even put it between your fingers. You will stop and stare at it, and then ask yourself, 'Is this really what I want to do?'"

3. The Secretary—Gorgeous but Obese

You may hold the opinion that fat is funny. It is no accident that Santa Claus, with his good-natured "Ho-ho-ho," has a big round belly. Fat people are stereotyped as having a sense of humor, of being non-worriers and being easy to live with. Once you see a seventy-pound-overweight man struggle to do a simple task such as rising from a chair or the more difficult task of breathing, once you see such a man weep as he describes his inability to function at his work, to perform sexually, or to participate in any kind of sports, fat is no longer funny.

The situation, if anything, is even worse for the woman forty or fifty pounds overweight. She is aware that people giggle at her, sometimes behind her back, sometimes brutally to her face. She is the butt of jokes intended to be funny but are in reality harsh. She too has difficulty functioning at her job, participating in sports, dancing, or sexual activity.

Making a fetish of being slim for esthetic reasons, as is done in many countries, including our own, is to be condemned. Some men and women who dread becoming obese go to the other extreme to achieve thinness, believing that being skinny is attractive. My chief concern about being obese or being a skeleton is the matter of health. People who disavow sensible nutritional necessities in order to become thin will sooner or later begin to suffer malnutrition and kindred ailments. Those who allow themselves to become obese are also in danger of developing serious health conditions such as varicose veins, heart disease, and brain damage—not to mention the painful condition which develops in feet and legs.

I saw the Broadway hit play *My Fat Friend,* starring Lynn Redgrave, and laughed my head off—superb acting and hilarious punch lines, one a minute. At the play's beginning Miss Redgrave is about fifty pounds overweight. She has a brief encounter with a solid, straight man who is on his way to the airport, leaving the country on a five-month work assignment for his firm. He liked her; they were together a day and a night. Lynn has two men boarding at her house, neither of them interested in women. The older man chides and browbeats her into losing weight. The nice-looking man will return at Christmas. If he is greeted by a tall, slim, beautiful woman, perhaps he will . . .

The idea takes hold, Lynn goes on a vigorous crash diet, plus strenuous daily exercises. She loses the fifty pounds. As promised in his letters from abroad, the man she knew for a day and a night returns at Christmas. Lynn Redgrave has never appeared more beautiful. At the end of the play she is slim with a charming coiffure and wearing beautiful clothes. The climax of the play is that the solid, straight eligible man is astonished and disappointed at what he sees; he rejects her because she no longer is flabby fat. He will not offer her friendship or marriage or even the bed. He leaves her immediately and the play is downhill from that point. The finale is within a few minutes. The audience no longer laughs uproariously; it belches but does not laugh. The reason: even humorous fiction must have at least a speck of resemblance to reality or it becomes hopeless slapstick or nauseating surrealism. The reality is obvious: a trim, youngish man of intelligence and virility will have difficulty relating to a woman who crushes him in bed.

If such unreality is true of the fat woman and the trim man, it is just as true with a slim woman and a paunchy man. There is one exception: women endure the indignities of the crushing, panting, obese male with far more patience than vice versa. Up to the present society has conditioned and reconditioned the woman by giving her few options . . . but "times are changing, times are changing."

Maria, who came to me for help, was thirty-six years of age; she looked like a woman in her late forties. She was 5 feet 6 inches tall and weighed 200 pounds. "What in the name of God will become of me? I've tried Weight Watchers, every crash diet on the market, from pills to protein and water. My doctor says there is absolutely no glandular imbalance. Speaking of the doctor, following the last examination, he looked at me and said in a very serious tone, 'Your trouble is food.' In spite of my misery, his profound statement cracked me up."

"Describe for me your eating pattern . . . from morning till bed-time."

"I keep lying to myself: 'I don't eat as much as Hazel and yet Hazel doesn't get fat.' That's a lie. . . . I know it but I keep saying it. I eat between meals. I eat like a horse before going to bed. I eat three enormous meals a day. I eat when I'm not hungry. I eat when I'm full to the chin. I drink wine, beer, and liquor as much as my paltry salary will allow or as much as I can con from my friends. I hide chocolate bars and cookies from my mother; this can get messy in the summer months."

"What, besides pounding the typewriter and eating, do you do?" She was a secretary-typist in a large publishing house.

"For several years, I forced myself into a variety of activities, such as dancing, then the clubs and bars for singles, then arts and crafts. I took tennis lessons, thinking that if I learned to play I might lose some of the weight and also I might meet a guy who would feel comfortable being seen with me. I didn't finish the ten lessons. Some of the players, men and women, giggled and laughed when I tried to run after the ball, and I could not take it. So I quit. Now I go to work, agonize through eight hours, come home, and eat. I haven't had a date in four years . . . started putting on loads of weight five years ago."

With great effort she shifted her weight on the couch, then said, "Will you agree to try to help me?"

Word in certain circles had gotten around that I would not see a compulsive eater. There was an element of truth in this: the compulsive eater is one of the most difficult people to work with. Characteristics are similar to those of the alcoholic, plus two additional features: First, food is an acceptable part of our way of life. Everywhere one turns in our society there is a meal, coffee break, or snack. It is considered bad manners if you do not eat food the hostess has prepared. Being on a diet is not a good excuse; you can break your diet just once. Second, the compulsive eater must continue to eat to live. The alcoholic is not simply a heavy drinker; he is one who, when he takes the first drink, continues to drink until he is sloppy drunk. The alcoholic in a sense is always an alcoholic. He can never be a "social" drinker; one cocktail or one beer and then he drinks until the lights go out. However, the compulsive eater cannot be taken off food! He must continue to eat and eating feeds his compulsion!

I had known Maria since she was a child. The family moved East about the same time as I did, and in a superficial way we had kept in touch. Maria at age twenty won a beauty contest. It had been eight years since I last saw her. In that time she was divorced, fired from a public relations job, and had put on forty or fifty pounds. I would not have recognized her except for the striking blond hair, the lovely face, a dimple in the right cheek, and a smile that could light up a room. I agreed to see her provided she would meet three conditions: First, she would agree to a minimum of ten hypnotic sessions scattered over twenty weeks. Second, on her own she would make an effort to eat low- rather than high-caloric food. Third, she would borrow money—perhaps from her mother—and enroll for six months in an exercising class where there were professional instructors.

She agreed. That very day we began the first hypnotic session. I used the same method of induction with Maria as I had with Bob, the alcoholic, and Gino, the cigarette addict. It was lengthy, but it produced a deep-level hypnotic state where a subject would be responsive to strong posthypnotic suggestions. When she reached her lowest level, I began the application; I had already decided on the direction the suggestion would take. This is the way it went:

"Maria, from toes to head, your body is completely relaxed, the tension has been drained off. You have complete freedom to accept or reject the exercise I shall now give you."

She mumbled sleepily, "I accept."

"You must use your imagination. . . . In front of you is a huge color television set. It has double doors covering the screen. Nod your head if you can see the set clearly."

She nodded.

"Now, slowly open the doors and turn the set on. The picture you see will be in bright, clear color and it will show one of the most memorable events in your life. As soon as the picture becomes clear tell me what you see."

She paused for several seconds and whispered, "It's the Miss America pageant . . . all the girls . . ."

If she had said something else, I would have let her describe her first picture, then I would have given a suggestion relating to the beauty pageant or perhaps I would have asked a direct question. But the latter was not necessary—the most memorable event in Maria's life was winning the pageant. Some people, and I am one of them, feel that to attach importance to an exploitative and superficial experience such as a beauty pageant is one of today's tragedies. Not so with Maria—it was the greatest event in her life.

"What are you and the girls doing?"

"We're walking down the runway in bathing suits."

"Can you see *yourself* clearly?"

"Yes, clearly."

"Describe Maria for me, including weight and dimensions."

Her voice choked a little as she began, "I am tall and slim, my hair looks so beautiful, I am smiling . . . not a plastic smile, I'm really smiling."

"Can you see the dimple?"

"Oh, yes."

"Continue."

"My walk is graceful. . . . I look wonderful in the bathing suit."

"Give me your exact dimensions."

She started to weep, tears trickled down both cheeks.

"Crying will be good for you. . . . Take this tissue." I keep a box of tissues in the counseling room for occasions such as this. She reached for it, continued to weep and to wipe the tears away. I waited and said, "Take your time. When you feel better, you may continue."

Within minutes she answered my question concerning her dimensions; the tears were almost gone. She said, "My bust, 37 inches; waist, 29 inches; weight, 124 pounds . . . height, 5 feet 6 inches."

"You won the contest, didn't you?"

The tears were gone. "Yes, yes, I did."

"Were you extremely disappointed when you failed to win at Atlantic City?"

"More than that . . . it broke me up; I was positive I would be selected as Miss America. Do you remember what I did in the talent division?"

"I'm sorry. . . . I can't recall."

"Baton twirling. . . . I don't think the judges like baton

twirlers. I got some prizes for winning the state contest, but I quit college, went to a commercial school."

"Before you turn the set off, the cameras will zoom in on you . . . a good, strong picture of a girl with the dimple and the perfect figure. All right, the cameras begin to move. Lift your right hand when only *your* picture is on the screen."

Within seconds she lifted her hand.

"The girl you see on that screen is you, Maria; as you were then, you will be again. Pause for just a moment. Turn the set off and close the doors."

"It's off. The picture is gone."

"No, Maria, the picture is gone from the set, but it is not gone from your mind."

While she was still in the trance, I closed the session by reviewing the three conditions we agreed to: a minimum of ten sessions, she would eat low- rather than high-caloric foods, she would enroll in an exercise class. Then I said, "You did not put on this weight in three months; you will not take it off in three months. Our hypnotic sessions will not only increase motivation; they will also create within you patience and confidence to a degree which you have never before possessed."

Slowly she came out of the trance. I rarely say the first word when a subject opens his eyes. Her eyelids had become extremely heavy and she had difficulty opening them. When they finally opened she sat quietly. I waited. At last she looked at me and said, "I can do it."

Twenty weeks went by. Maria stuck to the three requests I had made. Immediately she began to lose weight: the first week, the loss was five pounds; then it tapered off until she was losing an average of two or three pounds a week, so that by the time the hypnotic sessions ended she had lost fifty-four pounds. Her figure was stunning, the smile was even more attractive. "Ten more to go," she said. "With all the rewards I've gotten, nothing will ever again make me put on weight. . . . I have a confession to make to you."

"I hear confessions all the time. What's yours?"

"The first three weeks, I almost went out of my mind, but I didn't want you to know. I couldn't sleep, I became constipated, and often I literally had to run from food. I believed then and I know now that had it not been for hypnosis, I would never have had the strength to turn away from food offered so freely."

Then she made an announcement: "My mother is a wonderful human being; however, I'm leaving the house in Riverdale and taking a job back in the old home town . . . the same firm with the same job I had before coming to New York."

I congratulated her. We were standing; she was ready to leave. Suddenly she moved forward, kissed me full on the lips, and then said, "I love you very much, and have for all these weeks we've worked together."

With considerable effort, I retained my composure. Before I could say anything, she ran from the room, looked back once, smiling and waving as she left.

I sat in the large chair thinking back over the weeks I had worked with Maria. Her confession, I decided, was not limited to the first three weeks of anguish. Though keeping it cleverly disguised, I think now, she fell in love with me. Her love for me and wanting desperately to gain my respect for her were more powerful than the hypnosis. This was something more than "transference."

Two weeks later her mother called me and through bitter tears cried, "Maria left this morning alone for Pittsville; she bought an old car and was so happy. She crashed on the Pennsylvania Turnpike. . . . Now my beautiful baby is dead."

I don't quite remember, but I choked and said, "Oh, God, what irony."

I was still dazed as her mother continued, "When funeral arrangements are made, the family will be pleased if you conduct the service for her."

I managed to say, "Of course, I will. . . . Just let me know."

IV

Hypnotic Anesthesia

1. A Psychiatrist Experiences Hypnotic Anesthesia

Dr. Ann Keil is one of New York's outstanding psychiatrists. She came to my office in early 1974 struggling with a genuine case of cigarette addiction. Dr. Keil was a responsive subject. With five sessions the addiction was broken and the lingering nightmare urges for cigarettes were lessened. She discovered firsthand that hypnosis has within itself the seeds of its own strength, and this can be communicated to the person in such a way that incentive is increased, strength added to the will, and unconscious motivation toward the desired goal realized.

Dr. Keil, as it is with so many of us, has a low threshold of pain, especially where the dentist is concerned. She, like myself, becomes a white-knuckle patient while sitting in the dentist's waiting room. On a recent occasion a tooth required attention, a filling, with needle injection of the gum, the drill—the works. The thought of the needle injection with the burring of the drill was too much. She told her dentist about the experience she had with hypnosis in my office several months previously. "Fine," the dentist said. "I'll tell you precisely what to do. Close your eyes for a moment, try to re-create the exact feelings you experienced when you were in Dr. Shrader's office. Take a moment and reflect. I'm sure you'll soon be relaxed and we can fill the tooth without anesthesia, and furthermore, your gums will become numb, completely resistant to any pain."

She closed her eyes for several moments, re-created the scene in my office, and experienced again that pleasant sensation of total relaxation. She nodded her head to the dentist. He began drilling the tooth, and from beginning to end there was no pain. Dr. Keil says she could feel the touch of the drill but positively no pain whatsoever.

I'm inclined to believe that the dentist is a better hypnotist than I! He knew exactly the right thing to say and it worked.

Question: What can be done to convince men and women in the healing professions that there need be no stigma attached to the use of hypnosis, that hypnosis can become a useful tool in their hands? For many years in this country almost anyone connected with hypnotism has been considered a charlatan or a con artist. Considering the thousands of physicians, dentists, surgeons, obstetricians, psychiatrists, psychoanalysts, counselors, only a fraction of a per cent recognize hypnosis as an aid in their work.

Hypnosis is waging the same battle as acupuncture, except that it has been battling for many more years in this country. James Reston of the New York *Times* may have his appendix removed in China with acupuncture and without chemical anesthesia. He may tell his doctor friends back home; newspapers give the event headline treatment; still the resistance to acupuncture in most of the country is strong. In several states a curious condition exists: Physicians (M.D.) are being taught acupuncture by non-licensed but qualified men trained in this art. They permit these men to teach them, but will not permit them to use their skills on patients!

In 1965 and 1973, I made seminar trips to the Soviet Union. The first group was composed mainly of college professors, men and women. Since it was a seminar study group, conferences were arranged ahead of our arrival. We spent days in various universities (including the great University of Moscow), hospitals, and mental institutions. In each of these places we had access to the best men in their specialized fields. The duration of the first trip was five weeks. I had occasion to talk to a number of scientists, some of whom showed a mild interest in hypnosis, but less interest in related extrasensory perception. In fact, on one or two occasions when I raised the question I encountered from those in the academic community the same type of smug contempt as exists in this country.

Eight years later I returned to the Soviet Union. The trip was shorter, but I met and talked with a number of university people. Also, since it was winter and schools were open, I had greater access to young adults. I found both adults and young adults excited about hypnosis, especially anesthesia hypnosis. Russians were also interested in ESP—most of all in psychokinesis—in 1973. A physicist said to me (speaking perfect English), "In your country scientists are still trying to *prove* the validity of hypnosis, acupuncture, psychokinesis, etc. In our country we've passed the 'prove it to me' stage and are finding ways to make use of these *normal* experiences." It was a matter-of-fact statement from a professor of physics. His use of the word "normal" intrigued me. Here, when we refer to hypnosis, ESP, etc., we use the word "paranormal." I am sure there is still some resistance in Russia in the pursuit of these controversial fields, but I must admit that within a short period of eight years the climate had dramatically changed. Areas we now term "paranormal" are being accepted and applications of them are taking place on a wide scale.

In 1958 the American Medical Association formally approved hypnosis as a valid medical and dental tool and recommended that physicians familiarize themselves with its therapeutic uses. Since the AMA has spoken, the number of physicians and therapists using hypnosis has increased, but the increase has been marginal. Prior to 1958 there were no medical schools or psychology departments in any university in the country which made hypnosis a required course. Today there are several medical schools which require students to study the history, theory, practice, and application of hypnosis.

In many ways I have been impressed with the work done at the Menninger Clinic, Topeka, Kansas, which under expert leadership is willing to take a risk in fields where conservative universities hesitate. Notice that as far back as *1943* the *Bulletin of the Menninger Clinic* carried the following report:

> Among the experiments which have been made with forms of effective psychotherapy requiring less time and less training than psychoanalysis, one of the most promising would seem to be hypnosis. This powerful and dramatic method of treatment has long been neglected in psychiatry.

Progress has been made in the use of chemical anesthesia; however, it is well to remind ourselves that when a life is lost on an operating table the loss is due more often to the misuse or overuse of chemical anesthesia than a blunder on the part of the surgeon.

Since hypnotic anesthesia fascinates me more than any other area of hypnosis, the next four sections of this chapter will also deal with people in pain who found help in the power of hypnosis when they needed it.

2. The Actress with the Beard

Mary L. is one of those people who are objects of envy for the rest of us in the common herd. Just turned thirty, she possesses extraordinary talents in a variety of fields. She is a fashion model, a concert singer, and an excellent actress. Beyond all of this, she is beautiful—a young Ava Gardner.

At twenty-six she was in an automobile accident which nearly cost her her life. She was riding in the front seat of the car when the accident occurred. Her head went through the windshield and she was severely cut under the chin and up the right side of the face and temple. She was rushed unconscious to a nearby hospital. A plastic surgeon, who was joined by two other surgeons, performed a perfect operation on Mary's throat and face. Today, the throat scar under the chin can hardly be seen. The face scar is hidden by a head of lovely black hair.

For some reason, soon after the accident, Mary began to grow a heavy beard, especially under and above the chin.

The beard is black and very stiff (much fuller than mine). Of course, the beautiful one went without delay to an electrologist, who took a personal interest in the young actress. Immediately the electrologist ran into difficulty. Mary could not stand the pain of the electrologist's needle, especially when the needle went in near the scars. After three or four minutes, tears would come into her eyes and the electrologist would be forced to cancel the remainder of the time. Electrologists use a small needle which enters the face and goes to the root of each unwanted hair, one by one. Her hand controls the needle, the foot touches a floor pedal each time the needle enters the skin. In the majority of instances this procedure carries with it little pain; at least, most people can endure the pain for

fifteen or twenty minutes. Not so with Mary. The longest period of
time the electrologist could do her work was five to six minutes. At
this rate it would have taken years to clear the skin of the heavy
black hairs.

Through an actress friend, Mary heard about my work and
called for an appointment. In a preliminary interview she recounted
the above story and I in turn gave my evaluation of what hypnosis
might be able to do for her. At our second conference we went immediately into induction. Mary was so highly motivated that I
would have guessed her to be able to go into the deepest level.
However, the automobile had left scars other than those on her
face, and the pain resulting from the electrologist's needle created
unconscious resistance. However, she proved to be a medium
responsive subject, which permitted numbness to be produced so
that she would feel no pain.

As soon as the subconscious took over, I gave Mary suggestions
that her right hand would become cool and then cold. She was to
imagine the hand being plunged into a bucket of ice water, remain-
ing there until it became numb. I then suggested that the left hand
would become warm, warmer, and then hot. She was to imagine
herself in front of an open fire, the left hand sufficiently near to pick
up heat. I took Mary's right hand (the cold one) and began to rub
slowly two fingers. "When I reach the count of three, these two
fingers will grow numb. The numbness will last for nearly one hour
from the time you leave this office." Then I took the numbed fingers
and gently forced them to rub the back of her left hand (the hot
one). "Now, Mary," I said, "you will rub the back of your left hand
in a small circle. Gradually, that spot will become cold and numb
simply because you have touched it with your numb fingers. I shall
count to three, the numbness will have set in . . . one . . . two
. . . three. With the nails on the fingers of my right hand I will dig
into the numb spot and stop short of drawing blood. If you feel only
the touch of my fingers, do not lift your right hand. If you feel pain,
lift the right hand immediately." I dug my fingers into the numb
spot on Mary's left hand. Harder and harder. No pain. Marks were
left but no pain. Then I said, "You will go directly from my office
to your electrologist [three short blocks away]. When you first lie on
the table, touch the scars under the throat and on the side of the

face with your two numb fingers. Whatever spots you touch will instantly become numb, and as I said, the numbness will last approximately one hour."

She came out of the hypnotic state smiling. "I wouldn't have believed your nails went into my hand, but I see the marks, and besides, my two fingers, right here, feel numb."

She hurriedly left the office. The electrologist was waiting. She lay on the table, and before the needle entered her face the first time, she began to rub the sensitive areas of her throat and face. Malvina, the electrologist, thought this procedure a little strange. But Mary said, "Go ahead. Take as much time as you can give me." She proceeded for about twenty-five minutes, and could not believe how much of the face she was able to treat. "What on earth?" she exclaimed. Mary told her the story. Malvina had to see the process as it was done. The next time Mary visited the electrologist, the hypnotic process was demonstrated in her office for one who felt that such a thing could not be done. It was as effective the second time as the first.

Mary's visits to my office lengthened. I saw her over a period of six months. Today, the talented one is more beautiful than ever.

3. An Aging Man with a Non-diagnosable Pain

Tom, fifty-seven, has been a personal friend for a number of years. His wife, Martha, is a charming woman. Throughout a long marriage they have continued to be genuinely devoted to each other. All of us were distressed when Tom had to retire from a lucrative business (a chain of ice-cream outlets) which he had developed from the ground floor. He made money, invested wisely so that he and his wife can live comfortably the rest of their years. Money can do many things for us; however, there are times when, with the best of specialized care, it cannot bring us good health.

For the past two and a half years, my friend has been in excruciating pain which is localized inside the right groin above the knee on a direct line across from the testicles. During this time he was, of course, treated by his family physician, Dr. John K., who then referred him to a number of specialists. Tom has been seen and examined by eleven specialists, including a psychiatrist. He has been hospitalized for weeks at a time. Phlebitis was considered but tests revealed no trace. X rays and biopsies for cancer were taken; the right thigh bone underwent a painful test for tuberculosis of the bone. He was given a battery of allergy tests which included foods, liquor, dust, feathers, cats, dogs, New York smog, etc., etc., etc. He lost forty pounds and went down to about 120 pounds. (He stands almost six feet.)

His family physician sent him home from the last hospitalization and decided to keep him as comfortable as possible with sleeping pills and pain killers. Tom was suffering from a non-diagnosable pain in the groin. One day the physician (this time on the telephone) said to Tom's wife, "We've tried everything else. I'm ready to recommend hypnosis. The pain is obviously psychosomatic, and there is a possibility that Tom could be helped." Martha responded, "I'm glad to hear you say that—I was afraid you would disapprove." The doctor retorted, "On the contrary, I think we should give it a try. Dr. C. is an analyst friend of mine who specializes in the use of hypnosis." Martha answered strongly, "Please do not mention Dr. C. to Tom. His brother went to him several months ago. His fees are exorbitant and he has a gruff, indifferent manner." (The brother was no worse, except that his bad temper has increased, and he now holds hypnotism and hypnotists in contempt. He was not helped, even in the slightest.) "Do you know anyone else you prefer to send him to?" the doctor asked. She replied, "Yes, a man with considerable experience, a clergyman who uses hypnosis in connection with his counseling program."

Martha has a sense of humor, and through all their troubles has retained it, at least to a degree. With a smile in her voice, she reconstructed this story to me the day of the telephone conversation with their physician, Dr. John K. The doctor was silent for what seemed an eternity. He started to speak but choked. Martha said that she thought he was having a heart attack. "John, are you all right?" He wheezed and said, "I'm all right. I just can't buy the idea of Tom going to a clergyman for hypnosis. Is the clergyman young, middle-aged, old? How much experience has he had?"

Martha described to the doctor something of my background, the research and practice I have been doing for more than a quarter of a century. Then she had a sensible idea. She gave the doctor the names of three people in New York who had come to me and were helped—a college professor, a fellow physician, and a housewife. The doctor, now recovered, said, "I'll get back to you sometime this evening." He then proceeded to call the people she mentioned.

About ten that night, the doctor called, "I'm convinced. Get Tom to your minister friend as quickly as possible."

Since Tom's brother had such a disappointing experience with hypnosis, he too was skeptical. "I know Wesley is a good guy—but I can't see that hypnosis could help what I've got."

Martha replied, "You tried acupuncture, the baths, a psychiatrist, eleven physicians. What do you have to lose?"

Tom got out of bed the next day. He and Martha came to my apartment, which was more convenient than the office. I had not seen Tom for a couple of months and was aghast at the weight loss and the thin, pale face.

"How's the pain today?" I asked.

"Bad—the pain killers are losing their strength." Without much delay I began a trial induction and gave him several hypnotic exercises. What does one do with a fifty-seven-year-old man who has been in constant pain for two and one half years, a pain that is nondiagnosable? Following the induction, I did not attempt direct pain-relieving suggestions. Instead, I explained to him, while he was still in the hypnotic state, that under hypnosis he would have no conception of *time* . . . for the reason that *time* was distorted. He could have been in the hypnotic state three minutes or an hour and would not have known the difference. "So, Tom," I said, "we shall distort the time element in the pain by using the telescope method. The pain will not be eliminated, but the time span between the pains will be lengthened. For instance, the power of the subconscious is so great that it will make you pain-free for seven consecutive hours. The pain will return, but its duration will be no longer than two minutes. Seven hours free from pain; two minutes of pain. Tomorrow, when I see you again, you will move into a deeper state of relaxation, tension will be relieved, and the time span between the pains will be retained."

I saw Tom five consecutive days, and then saw him for reinforcement once a week for two months. I doubt that the pain will ever disappear completely. Tom, for one reason or another, *needed* that pain. *He needed it desperately and was not going to give it up even if it killed him.* I am positive I know the reason for the pain, but I shall not confront Tom with it, and neither do I believe that letting him discover the reason for himself would "cure" him. There is a possibility that he would become worse. I am delighted that he immediately began to eat normally. He has gained fifteen pounds and moves about quite easily. Tom still does not know what has happened to him; he was sent home from the last hospital to die. It may be of some comfort to him to know that neither do I know what really happened.

The doctor's reaction to Martha's suggestion that Tom see a clergyman who practiced hypnosis in connection with counseling cases, raises an important question.

What kind of cases will I accept and what kind do I refuse? I refuse to take any person who gives the impression of being in a psychotic or near-psychotic condition. This includes schizophrenics, paranoid schizophrenics, and obvious manic-depressives. I have done considerable study in various branches of psychology, but one of the most helpful experiences occurred during my seminary years listening to lectures and visiting patients in the mental wards of the huge city hospital in Louisville, Kentucky. A half dozen students would enter a room (cell) with the professor from the medical school and a professor from the seminary. The medical professor would proceed to describe the condition of these patients, who were out of touch with reality. He would ask us to try not to show feelings such as revulsion or fear. Prior to entering a cell, the professor would explain the nature of the person's illness. For instance, he would say, "In this room is Mr. Jones, a schoolteacher for many years." He would then give us a biographical description of the man as well as the prognosis. Then he would say, "For the past three months Mr. Jones has been the Pope. As we enter his chambers he will climb on top of the radiator, his throne. Sometimes he never utters a word but other times he motions. This means he wants to bless us by laying his hands on our heads. Cooperate with him immediately; one at a time approach the radiator, kneel slightly, and permit him to touch you with his hands." (The first time I went through this ritual, I must confess I felt uncomfortable.)

It is not my practice to deal with psychotics who are out of touch with "our" world. However, every minister, counselor, hypnotist should have sufficient background that enables him to recognize the borderline psychotic.

I do not take people with deeply embedded neurotic trends. Such people, of course, are in touch with reality and to a certain extent can perform and relate. A neurosis is a "normal" function which has become highly exaggerated, is characterized by compulsion, and is accompanied by pain, often not localized. Such a person usually requires an enormous amount of time from the counselor, and I do not have enough time to devote to such work. One exception I have made in recent years is the case of Tom, reported above. He and Martha were my friends, and it was on this basis I agreed to see him.

I never see a person who is suffering from a *pain* unless he has been carefully checked by a physician and referred.

Cases of obesity must also be checked by a physician. If there is a disturbance of the thyroid or some other gland, hypnosis will not injure such a person, but it surely will not help him.

Cases where I do not hesitate to attempt aid:

Any type of symptom which is psychosomatic, such as Tom's pain described in this chapter. Here I must have a referral from a physician or psychoanalyst.

I see a limited number of alcoholics and drug addicts.

Cases involving anesthesia, with the restriction listed above.

The same is true with phobias, such as fear of flying.

Insomniacs are exceedingly difficult to help; however, by careful selectivity, I agree to work with a limited number of these frantic people.

People with certain sexual disturbances. Though not a hard-and-fast rule, I prefer working with couples rather than a single person.

Amnesia cases are a natural target for hypnosis. One may not secure all the information he desires and there are times when that which comes forth is distorted. However, years of experience is the tool which enables the hypnotist to separate fact from fantasy.

The stutterer is as difficult to work with as the alcoholic or the insomniac. I see a limited number of such people.

Listless, withdrawn, "no reason to live" people often respond to the hypnotic process. Some in a remarkably short time.

Cigarette addiction. I rarely turn down anyone hooked on cigarettes. For years I have crusaded to help as many people as possible to become unhooked from that innocent piece of white poison. I am convinced that cigarettes are among the most dangerous addictive drugs in our society. The slow, suffocating manner in which the addict dies is painful to contemplate much less watch.

In the next section I deal, in the hypnotic process, with pain that has seeped into the deepest recesses of the psyche. It is more difficult to reach than physical pain and for the sufferer much more difficult to endure.

4. The Rejected—How to Kill the Pain

Most of the people I see on a one-to-one basis are either coming out of, or just entering, a disastrous love affair. Rachel was just coming out of such a relationship. In her middle thirties, she had been married five years, divorced, and had her fling. Then she met Bart. Of her former husband she said bitterly, "He was cold, detached, stubborn, selfish, sexless, and stupid." Of Bart she said, "He was a beautiful person . . . warm, interested in me, flexible, tremendous in bed, and brilliant." Bart was on the faculty of one of the colleges in the City University System; he taught psychology.

She sighed and wiped away the tears. "He was the handsomest man I ever knew, his big blue eyes haunt me, the thought of his touch makes me weak, his body was like that of a Greek god." Bart had never been married; he was a few years older than Rachel.

When she first started coming for counseling, she asked me, "Did you ever meet Bart?" Being in academic circles virtually all my life, it was not an unlikely question. I said that I had met him. Then she asked, "What do you think? . . . Isn't he everything I described?"

I did not get the connection between Bart T. and the man Rachel described. True, he was a tall, handsome man, but in every way his insecurities showed through—overdressed, arrogant, narcissistic, or, as we say, "in love with himself." He suffered from verbal diarrhea, and though not stupid, he was not a well-informed man. He had failed his graduate exams twice, and though Rachel did not know it, he was finished at the college come next year. The last time I saw Bart he told me that college teaching—at the instructor level—was not paying him enough money to live on. He was leaving the faculty next June to become an advertising salesman. My answer to Rachel's question was short of a lie. "Bart is a handsome man. The few times I met him I found him interesting."

The romance between Rachel and Bart had begun about six months before she came to me for help. She had been no bar pickup or a singles-club pigeon. They had been properly introduced by Rachel's brother-in-law. It was a week of fascinating dating before he kissed her. It was a month before he invited her to Bermuda for a weekend with him. As yet Rachel and I had not reached hypnosis. We were in a counseling situation. I let her talk and talk and talk. She described in detail that weekend in Bermuda. It was the most heavenly thing that had ever happened to her. He wined her, dined her, sexed her, and filled her full of humorous stories about himself.

When they returned to New York, they continued to see each other (and no one else) about three times a week, including every weekend. Rachel held a high-paying, monotonous job in data processing, but looking forward to being with Bart made her work less of a drudgery. She made more money than he, so she insisted on picking up her share of the tab when they went to the theater or a concert or a high-priced restaurant. Two months went by, then three, then four months. Rachel was on cloud nine. They never discussed marriage. Though she had sworn that she would never get locked into marriage again, she would have married Bart at a day's notice. Both of them appeared to be thriving on the relationship. One night as they lay in bed in her Upper East Side apartment, relaxed by lovemaking and several glasses of wine, Rachel said, "Bart, it's silly for us to keep two apartments. Why don't you move in with me, or I'll move in with you." (I suspected that hers was much the nicer apartment.)

He raised himself on an elbow, turned up the table light, lit a cigarette, and said, "For the past couple of weeks I've wanted to have a heart-to-heart talk with you. The proper time never presented it-self. . . . There is no proper time, I suppose."

Rachel went cold. By the tone of his voice, she knew something serious was about to happen. She moved off the bed, reached for a negligee, and sat in a chair facing him. He continued. "This relationship has ended. . . . For me it has been one of the best, certainly it has lasted longer than the others. I have never been able to be with a woman in a steady relationship longer than three months, and most of the women I have been with had to be under twenty-five. I guess you would call that a hang-up."

Rachel was nearly his own age, a little on the plump side, but as she was about 5 feet 7 inches, the plumpness was not so evident. She was speechless. He was walking out on her just like that. Through tears she asked in a trembling voice, "You mean I shall never see you again?"

"I don't think we should see each other again. . . . Only by chance shall we meet and then as strangers."

He arose from the bed, went to the washroom, dressed, leaned down, kissed her forehead, and left.

"When it happened," she said, "I thought I had been dreaming. . . . In one form or another I had dreamed of losing him. But then I would wake up and remember that we were seeing each other that night."

I then asked Rachel, "Tell me again . . . how long has it been since the break?"

"Six months, two weeks, and three days."

She told me that she observed the anniversary of the night he first kissed her. Each week, Friday, she put a special rose on her lonely table as a remembrance of a love that had given her something to live for.

"I've tried everything I know to get him out of my mind . . . went to France for two weeks, tried dating other men . . . it was nauseous. I have taken special courses not related to my work, I joined a photographer's class, a weight-reducing program, a lecture series, an early-morning hiking group, and finally I've been bird watching. But I can't get the son of a bitch out of my mind."

"You can begin by eliminating the empty ceremony of the rose each Friday night."

"Actually, I quit that two weeks ago—the pain got worse."

"Give it a little time. . . . Perhaps you'll meet someone who will return your love in kind."

She looked at me as if to say, "Oh, yeah," but instead she said, "Do you think hypnosis could help me get rid of him?" Before I could answer she continued: "All of this gabbing we've been doing hasn't helped."

I said firmly and confidently, "We can get rid of him."

"How . . . what do we do?"

"It's easy . . . we can kill him."

"You mean hypnosis can make me *think* he's dead?"

"Not exactly . . . but hypnosis can erase Bart from your mind as if he had never existed."

"Let's get started now," she begged.

"I'd rather not. . . . Think about it for one more week . . . then if you want him erased, we will erase him."

The next week she came in, heavy with Bart on her mind but eager to get rid of him. The induction went well. Before we had completed the five deep breaths, she entered a medium-level trance. By the time we reached the stage of the "breathing of sleep," Rachel had relaxed, tension gone. For the first time in months she was at peace.

While she was still in the trance, I gave her an exercise. It went like this: "In your mind, you must visualize a huge blackboard. You are standing before it with a piece of chalk in your hand. Now write the numbers slowly from one to ten . . . all right, one, two, three, four, five, six, seven, eight, nine, ten . . . put the chalk down, pick up an eraser, and erase number six. Completely and neatly erase the number six. Rachel, have you followed me, have you done as I suggested? If so, lift your right hand." She lifted her right hand.

"Now count from one to ten. When you come to the number six you will not be able to say it . . . it's gone, you will not be able to articulate number six. Begin the count and make a strong effort to say 'number six.'" She began the count slowly. When she reached five, she stumbled; number six would not come out.

"If you cannot say 'six,' skip to seven and continue."

She began the count at seven and continued.

"Now try it one more time, this time a little faster. When you stumble at six, go immediately to seven." She came to six, could not say it, and continued on to seven, eight, nine, ten.

She was still in a deep trance and I said with authority, "You have erased the number six from your mind. It is no longer there. What you did with that number, you will now do with Bart. Number six represents the man you thought loved you. As you erased the number, so is he now being erased from your thoughts, your heart, your life, your interests. If ever again you think of him, it will be an act of recalling a stranger fleetingly known."

Her face, instead of being filled with anguish and pain, was a picture of peaceful serenity.

"Rest for a moment, let that which we have done sink deep in your mind. Ponder it, drink it in, accept it as fact. . . . Now I shall count to five; the number six will return to your vocabulary but Bart will not. Keep your eyes closed until the count has been completed. When your eyes open, your mind will become bright and clear. You will remain relaxed and at peace with yourself." I counted to five; she had some difficulty opening her eyes. I said, "Take your time, no hurry, take a little breath, you may want to stretch." With that her eyes slowly opened. She sat still for several minutes, nothing but silence in the room. She was relaxed; I was relaxed. I waited for her to speak. Finally she said, "I feel so peaceful."

So it was with Rachel. Bart became a stranger in one hypnotic session! She returned to my office several times, mostly for reinforcement. She left her data-processing job and took a position as a film editor. It has been more than a year since I have seen Rachel. She called last month and said, "Just checking in to say that all goes well. I now accept the bitter with the sweet."

5. A Baby Is Delivered

Of all the case studies in this book, this one is the only one for which I regret not being able to use the true names and places. But, for reasons best known to myself, this cannot be done.

Many years ago, I was living and working in an ultraconservative community. I was well acquainted with all of the doctors who were practicing there. There was not a psychiatrist in town, but there was a lovely new but small hospital. My physician friend Dr. B. stopped by late one evening and explained to me the situation with which he was confronted. A young couple three years before had moved from Connecticut and Dr. B. was Mrs. J.'s gynecologist. At this time she was two months pregnant and was excited about it and of course wanted him to deliver the baby. "They have a son, four. Now they are expecting a second child. They've told me they do not care if the child is a girl or another boy. *They want two children.*" The first child was delivered in Connecticut with hypnosis as the only anesthesia. The wife was a quiet, frail person who had a history of slight cardiac disturbances and also had a bout with tuberculosis some years previous. The Connecticut obstetrician used hypnosis with all of his pregnant patients who requested it and who were in a level sufficiently deep to produce complete anesthesia. This first experience of the frail one had been so highly successful that she and her husband thought it best that chemical anesthesia should be avoided if anything else could be used. "Natural childbirth" was a possibility; however, though some women are able through breathing exercises and the proper use of muscles to reduce pain to a remarkable degree, still a high percentage reduce it to a minimal level and tough it out by "biting the nail." Still others who attempt natural childbirth carry through the delivery until pain becomes so intense that chemical anesthesia must be used.

Neither the husband nor his wife wanted this second baby delivered in any way but by hypnosis.

Dr. B. that evening looked at me and with great earnestness in his voice said, "I know you cannot, in the months that are left, teach me enough about hypnosis to deliver this baby. I am totally ignorant of the process, yet several women whom I have delivered have had the same pleasant experience as Mrs. J. So I wondered if you would assist me in this pregnancy. . . ." Then he stammered, "You know how the people are in this community and at the hospital. If they thought the woman was being hypnotized, all hell might break loose." I remained silent; he had more to say. "Wes, is there any way you could get her ready, prepare her for the delivery, and be in the delivery room with her and with me when the time comes?"

Being a clergyman in that small town, I was taking as much of a risk as he, but the case presented a challenge. I said, "If Mrs. J. is a responsive subject, it can be done, and if you want me in the delivery room with you, I'll be there."

Dr. B. asked, "What do we do first?"

"Tell Mrs. J. and her husband to be in my office tomorrow at noon. I'll give her a few exercises, and then let you have the word whether or not I'll condition her for the delivery."

Mrs. J. and her husband came to the office promptly at noon the next day. I had met the couple on several social occasions. He taught history in the local high school, and our meetings had something to do with the school. Mrs. J. was far from being a beautiful woman, but I have never seen seen a face more angelic and more radiant than hers when she started talking about her pregnancy. She had had one miscarriage just a year previous. But she smiled with sweet determination as she said, "We want this baby very much." Her husband nodded and said, "We most certainly do."

Mrs. J. told me about her previous experience in childbirth with hypnosis, and what a surprising, pleasant event it was. A woman who gives birth under hypnosis is aware of everything that is taking place; she hears the physician's voice, she can obey his suggestions concerning breathing, using the muscles, etc. Furthermore, she is aware of the actual moment when the baby leaves the uterus and makes the journey down the canal and out into this strange world. If she were an excellent subject, the entire pelvic area would be anesthetized.

After a brief conversation the process was begun. I suggested that her hands would be cool and then cold. They became so in seconds. I then suggested that her hands would be warm and then hot. They reached the point of being hot in less time than it had taken for the suggestion of "cold."

"Now," I said, "Mrs. J., I will anesthetize a sensitive area of your right foot, the Achilles tendon." (Strong pressure here can make a person wince or scream in a matter of seconds.) I reached down and began to rub my fingers over the back part of the foot, just above the heel. "When I reach the count of three your heel will begin to grow numb." I slowly counted to three. Then I said, "Now one more time. When I reach the count of three this time, your heel will be completely numb, so numb that you will feel no pain, no matter how severely the heel is pinched." I dug my nails into the heel, deeper and deeper until I almost drew blood. Mrs. J. felt nothing.

She remained under the power of hypnosis for a few moments. "You are an excellent subject," I said. "Twice each month until the time of delivery you will be conditioned. By mere suggestion and without touching you any place, except the forehead, your body will be anesthetized."

Mrs. J. was in a state of exhilaration when she was brought into the conscious state, and exclaimed, "Oh, my God, it was just like before. I felt just like before!"

The husband had choked up and tears were in his eyes. "I know it'll be all right," he whispered.

Twice each month through the eighth, I met Mrs. J. in her obstetrician's office. We went through the same procedure. She became anesthetized by suggestion and touching her forehead. At the beginning of the ninth month, I explained to her exactly what would take place when heavy labor began. I would be in the room with the doctor. I said, "When he gives me the signal, there will be no verbalized form of induction. I will gently touch your forehead and whisper to the count of five. The count will be virtually inaudible but you will hear my voice. When I reach the count of five, your body, including stomach muscles and the entire region of the vagina, including the area of the uterus, will be anesthetized as if you had been given Demerol or morphine. Do you understand me, Mrs. J.?" She nodded her head and said, "Yes."

I wish there were a dramatic ending to this story, but there isn't. When the time came I went with Dr. B. to the hospital. Frail Mrs. J. looked at us and smiled. Labor had started; within less than an hour the doctor signaled to me. I went through the procedure described above, my hand on her head while whispering one, two, three, four, five. It was not long until the little one, a girl, made her entrance into this world. And it was accomplished without forceps, without chemical anesthesia, and without pain to the mother or baby.

The nurses in the delivery room were positive that Mrs. J. had used some form of natural childbirth. As I left the room to remove gown and gloves, I heard one of them say, "Reverend Shrader is such a good man; she might not have made it."

The other nurse replied, "Did you notice how he touched her forehead and whispered a prayer? He's a spiritual man."

They were impressed that I was willing to remain through the delivery. However, they overstated my "spirituality," even though they were correct in believing that I had offered a prayer in Mrs. J.'s behalf. There are more ways to pray than one. Dr. William E. F. Werner, gynecologist and obstetrician, in 1968 wrote in the *New York State Journal of Medicine* a significant statement concerning childbirth and hypnosis: "Since the science of obstetrics came into being we have been looking for a method to deliver mothers of healthy infants in a comfortable state. I feel that with delivery under hypnosis we can attain these goals."

Leslie M. LeCron writes in *The Complete Guide to Hypnosis,* "What are the advantages found in the use of hypnosis [in childbirth]? The most important is not for the mother but for the child. It is the only method entirely free of danger to the baby. As has been mentioned previously, use of any drug also affects the baby and its respiration is depressed when it is born. The baby born while the mother is in hypnosis is not drugged and almost invariably takes its first breath spontaneously, without the necessity of any stimulus. Such babies are found to be more healthy, cry less, feed better, and are more contented.

"For the mother the ability to have her baby with little or no pain is, of course, most desirable. Under hypnosis some women are able to shut off pain completely. Others feel pain but the threshold has been raised so it is not severe. With some, pain persists and drugs must be used. Even in this situation the anesthetist finds a much smaller amount of drug is necessary if the woman is in hypnosis. This is of value to both the mother and the baby.

"Statistics show that the time in labor is reduced when hypnosis is used. This seems to be about 20 per cent with a woman having her first baby. Those who have previously had a child usually are in labor a shorter time but this is further cut through hypnosis.

"Another advantage is that there is less postnatal shock. The amount of bleeding can be controlled and the healing process greatly speeded up. Hospital stay (now very expensive) is shortened one to three days."

V

Passivity—the Most Prevalent Curse

She was forty years of age, looked thirty, was tall with a trim figure, and gave the impression of being a successful career woman. So she was. A middle-level executive working for a national magazine. Married to a man who drank too much and worked too little—a would-be actor. One child, a daughter, who was a senior in high school.

Marilyn's beautiful façade had been developed over the years. However, beneath the surface there was a person who had reached the end of the line, ready to crack at a moment's notice. Her immediate superior in the office was a man who took delight in bullying her. When he discovered that her withdrawn, fearful nature would not permit her to fight back, he humiliated her because of what she had done or had not done. Often he would give Marilyn an assignment and the next day reverse his decision or, worse still, deny that he had ever given any such assignment. He would yell and swear at her in the presence of fellow workers, some of whom disliked Marilyn because they interpreted her withdrawn disposition as being cold and unfriendly.

She had been with the magazine for almost two years. Her impressive appearance and intimate knowledge of the work helped her to secure this position, which paid much more than her previous job with a small women's magazine. But money was not the only reason she left her former position. As she related the pathetic story —which every analyst, minister, and counselor has heard hundreds of times—it developed that her former boss, a female and a bitch, had also made her life miserable. So she jumped at the chance to change jobs. To Marilyn it was a promotion in more ways than one. However, she had not counted on walking into a position where her chief responsibility would be to a sadistic, pathologically aggressive male!

Marilyn, of course, could not stand up to her handsome, sometime actor husband. Oddly, the husband had no real inner strength, no firmness, no assertiveness with anyone except his wife. She loved him and could not consider a separation or divorce. She also feared him. Often in the midst of his tirades and temper tantrums, mainly over money, he cowed her and on several occasions had slapped her with blows that brought redness to the face and festering wounds to her spirit.

Her daughter was an impudent, spoiled brat. For the most part, she had been reared by Marilyn's mother, a widow who lived with the family in Brooklyn Heights. Marilyn was no match for her mother or her daughter, just as she was no match for her husband or the man to whom she was responsible at work.

So familiar symptoms developed. Though intelligent and highly skilled, she was becoming a non-functioning, non-productive person, isolated from friends and social functions. Here was a lifeless, listless, unhappy soul who had drifted from one physician, psychiatrist, analyst to another. Coming to my office was a painful decision of last resort. Never had she thought she would reach the point of seeing a hypnotist! She came by appointment, and after describing some of the details of her desperate plight, she asked, "Can you help me?"

Not everyone is a cigarette addict, a compulsive eater, or a sexual cripple, but virtually everyone has in one way or another suffered from the character defect known as passivity or passiveness. It was Alfred Adler who gave us the concept of "inferiority complex" with all of its twisting implications. The man is but the child grown tall. From his earliest moments he knows what fear is: at first, a fear of falling, then of being alone, or perhaps a fear of the dark. The list is without end. The boy grows to manhood. His fears deepen. Making a living sometimes is a monstrous and monotonous struggle. He knows that feebleness, the mate of the aging process, awaits him. He is a part of Nature, which will inevitably do him in; he is a part of Society, which more often than not works against him. With his decline in the face of Nature's unrelenting power and Society's indifference or hostility, the child-man begins to retreat within himself, assured that he is inadequate for the world into which he was thrust. Thus it is that a large number of people move deeper and deeper into this state of fear and dread, and growing older they become more passive and withdrawn. As such they invite hostility from others.

Another group of people, by incredible overcompensations, make an effort to burst the chains that bind them. The result is disastrous to the individual and sometimes disastrous to the world. On a grand scale there is the image of Adolf Hitler, who as a youngster was the meekest of the meek. Stalin, insanely cruel to the time of his death, studied for the priesthood and in early youth was known as a mild and obedient child. On the gangster level both John Dillinger and Al Capone would be included in the passive-aggressive types. If we bring the roll call up to date, and if we can believe her parents' story of the shy and quiet little girl, and if we can trust the validity of the hard-faced young woman looking into a bank camera while holding people at bay with a shotgun, the name of Patty Hearst would also be included.

The list of those who move from passivity to aggression is not limited to the famous or infamous. It includes on a smaller scale housewives and career women, salesmen and executives, artists and actors, bus drivers (especially) and professional men and women, many of whom literally clawed their way to the top of their world.

The list is longer of those who move from passivity to deeper passivity (Marilyn) until they become putty in the hands of those who wittingly or unwittingly destroy what little strength was once possessed. Such battered people lose their identity and become ghosts walking silently through fearful days.

The opposite of passivity is not pathological aggression or aggression itself. (Webster's defines aggression as "an unprovoked attack or an act of hostility.") The opposite of passivity is assertiveness, and this description must be preceded by the adjective *healthy*. When any person among us develops a personality whose dominant trait is *healthy assertiveness,* he has discovered the pearl of great price. This is the person who knows who he is, is aware of his strength and weakness, and is in touch with his feelings. He accepts without peacock pride or devastating loathsomeness his own self-image. He does not deliberately provoke a confrontation, nor will he, with tail between his legs, back away from an encounter, especially if there is an issue at stake. This is the person who moves firmly but speaks softly. He recognizes his own mortality (death) and accepts it without dread or fear. He does not yell, shout, or become profane in order to get his way. (I am weary with certain professional healers who confuse "talking it out" with yelling and lung screaming, which is supposed to exorcise sexual hang-ups, fears, guilt, and hostility. How lunatic can we, the healers, become?) The person who has refused to move from passivity to deeper passivity and who has been saved from the other extreme, that of clawing his way to meaningless aggression, is a person who has become assertive in the healthiest possible way. He is a person of reason, understanding, and granitelike strength.

"Can you help me?" Marilyn asked.

I looked at her carefully and in a confident voice said, "Through a series of hypnotic sessions you can be helped. Of this I am sure. Your personality will undergo certain changes for the better and you will discover a life style with which you can live."

It is necessary at this point to say something about treating symptoms rather than causes. Once it was held by a body of therapists that unless the *cause* of a flawed personality could be discovered, assimilated, and understood, the patient would never change for the better and certainly he could never be *cured*. For more than a score of years I have proceeded upon the principle enunciated so clearly in Dr. Lewis Wolberg's book *Hypnosis: Is It for You?* He writes: "By and large the time-honored dictum that symptoms removed by hypnosis must return in the same or substitute form or that the psychic equilibrium will be upset, precipitating a psychosis, is purely fictional. Relief can be permanent, and advantage may be taken of the symptom-free interlude to encourage a better life adjustment." Dr. Wolberg is joined in this point of view by such men as Dr. Joseph Wolpe, of Temple University, and a host of other non-Skinnerian behaviorists.

I once agreed to see a sixty-five-year-old man who had developed (learned) a phobia concerning elevators. For three years he walked up five flights of steps in his apartment building rather than use the elevator. I suppose that I, as a counselor, or an experienced analyst, could have spent five, eight, or ten years trying to dig out the cause —"why" the old man was afraid to ride an elevator. Such information may have been helpful, interesting, or even juicy. But the plain fact was that according to the statistical timetable, he did not have too many years left, and in just two hypnotic sessions, the aging subject was relieved of his fear of elevators. After the second session, I rode with him up and down several times. He was like a child at Christmas having great fun with a new toy. This experience occurred about four years ago. He is still alive, functioning, and reasonably happy.

Marilyn was in the group of those whose problem was symptomatic. The first set of instructions I gave to this shy, reserved person appears easy to perform, but to Marilyn it was as if I had asked her to walk down Fifth Avenue naked. In the second session, I suggested that for "homework" she would perform three tasks. No matter what happened, I told her to make an effort to keep cool.

"Have you ever made a reservation in a hotel on your own—not in writing but in person?"

"Never. I've had to work so consistently that I rarely get out of New York . . . so there would be no point."

"Here is your first assignment for the week. Go to a hotel, one of New York's better ones. Saunter up to the reservation clerk and calmly make a reservation for two, just for that night."

"What will the clerk think?"

"He will think you are a good-looking call girl who is entertaining an important man from distant parts just for the evening."

"Will he let me have the room?"

"Not if you choose one of three hotels I have in mind." I gave her the names of the three.

"I'll faint before I get out."

"No, you won't. We'll have a hypnotic session today. You will assert yourself as never before."

"But you said he won't give me the reservation on such short notice for one night. Is it because I am a single woman alone?"

"Both reasons, but in a positive way you are to *demand* a room. . . . You may be so persuasive that he will relent."

As I indicated, Marilyn's husband rarely worked, but she made an excellent salary and could afford the cost of the room. "If you get the reservation, invite your husband to an evening at one of the best."

"What next?"

"This one is a little easier, but not much. Tomorrow evening about 6 P.M. stand on the corner at Lexington and Fifty-fourth or Fifty-fifth for approximately five minutes. Watch for an attractive man, approach him, and say, "I'm sorry to bother you, but can you give me the correct time?""

"Oh, that's where some of the girls congregate for their night's work. . . . I couldn't."

"It will take a few minutes; there is nothing evil in asking a man or anybody else for the correct time."

"Suppose he misinterprets . . . and asks me to a bar."

"You are to smile sweetly and say, 'Really, all I wanted was the time of day.' At that hour, with the crowds, you will be safe. After you have approached the gentleman, hail a cab and you are done with him."

She was becoming more nervous by the minute. What next?

"This one requires no brashness, just plain assertiveness. Go to a bank where you're not known. At the loan department you tell Mr. Good Credit that you want to make a loan for fifteen thousand dollars. You need the money as quickly as possible. He will say, 'Are you married?' You will say, 'Yes.' He will say, 'Are you presently living together?' You will say, 'Yes.' He will say, 'For that kind of a loan we must have your husband's signature.' You will say, 'I do not want my husband to know about the loan.' He will say, 'What is your income?' You will give him the name of the magazine for which you work and the amount per annum. Mr. Good Credit will give you an application form to fill out, but he will also remind you that your husband must sign it. At this you become indignant. . . . 'Am I not a person in my own right?' etc., etc."

"Am I to make a scene?"

"If speaking firmly makes a scene, you will make a scene. Are you ready for a hypnotic session?"

"Yes . . . more than ready."

The induction of Marilyn was easy. She trusted me and responded beautifully: eyes closed for a few seconds . . . five deep breaths . . . suggestions concerning heaviness of head, eyelids, hands, and then the "breathing of sleep." At this point, I gave a posthypnotic suggestion: "That part of the mind, the subconscious, will emerge over both your conscious mind and your senses. Its power will reinforce you at the point of motivation, emotional strength, and confidence in yourself as a human being, as a woman in your own right, a person who can easily carry out the instructions I have given you . . . asking a hotel reservation clerk for a room for the night, asking a strange man on a busy street corner for the correct time, and confronting the manager of a bank loan department for a fifteen-thousand-dollar loan."

Within a few minutes she was out of the trance . . . her mind clear, her spirit confident, and her body relaxed.

"I believe I can do it," she said with determination.

Five days later she was back in my office to make a report on how she did with her assignments. "Which one did you find most difficult?" I asked. I thought she would say the first—asking for the hotel room. But no . . .

"The second. . . . There were two or three prostitutes walking up and down Lexington Avenue at the hour you mentioned. . . . I kept at least a half block from them. Then I saw him, a gentleman who came out of the Waldorf. . . . I went up to him and said, 'I'm sorry to bother you, but can you give me the correct time?' "

"What happened?"

"He looked at me for a moment, smiled knowingly, and said, 'Sure, it's five minutes after six.' "

"What did the gentleman do then?"

"Before I could say, 'Thank you,' he flagged a cab and was gone." She paused and said with a smile, "I don't think I would make a good prostitute . . . but it was a great experience, just to approach the man as I did. Without the session a few days ago, I don't believe I would have done that for a thousand dollars!"

"How'd you do at the bank?"

"It was a riot. . . . This tiny, bald-headed man appeared far more nervous than I. He took me into his office and said jerkily, 'What can I do for you?' I told him I wanted to make a loan. . . . I said, 'Interest rates are high, but I can give references, establish credit, and I'm sure I can meet the payments.' Then, exactly as you said, he began talking about the necessity of my husband's signature on the loan."

"How did you reply to that?"

"I told him my husband was a would-be actor whose income, above unemployment insurance, was a total of two thousand dollars per year. The banker had previously asked my income and I told him; he was sufficiently impressed. However, he insisted that I could not get the loan unless my husband countersigned it.

" 'Well,' he said, 'I guess that's that.' And began to shuffle some papers.

"Then I became assertive. . . . 'Wait one minute, sir. I know the laws of New York; I talked to my lawyer before coming here. *You* cannot deny me a loan if I can establish credit and if my income is sufficient to warrant it.' My tone was more than firm . . . it was hard. I said to myself, 'My God, are these *my* words?'

"The little man became more rattled than ever. Finally, he said, 'Here is an application form, fill it out, establish your credit, and return it to me. I can't promise the loan, but perhaps your application will be accepted.' . . . I took the paper and with my head up strode out of the bank."

I asked, "What about the hotel clerk and you?"

She blushed slightly but smiled and said, "It takes real nerve to be a call girl."

I looked closely at Marilyn and said to myself, "I had not noticed it before, but she's the image of a hundred-dollar-a-night call girl. She dresses well. She is extremely attractive. And without her shyness, she could be so cast!"

She gave me the name of the hotel . . . one of New York's finest. It was early afternoon when she entered it. "I went to the reservation clerk and said, 'My sister and her husband are coming into New York tonight, and they asked me to make a double-room reservation for them. They are now en route.'

"The clerk, in his captain's uniform, looked at me and sneered, 'We have no more rooms for tonight.'

" 'I don't believe you. . . . I've been standing here at least ten minutes. . . . Several single men, with no reservations, came by ~~d you gave each of them a room without a question.' I lifted my voice and said, 'I want to make a reservation for a room to-

night . . . tonight, I say, and if I don't get it, I demand to see the hotel manager immediately.'

" 'Why didn't one of them call and make their own reservation?'

"I replied, 'It's none of your business, but they called me from Chicago's O'Hare airport after trying several times to get through to you. I live in the neighborhood and thought it better, since it was short notice, to come in and explain the situation.'

"The clerk, unlike the bank manager, was unabashed and unnerved. He said, 'I'll let you talk to the manager.'

"He called first a young woman, who shook her head as if to say, 'I don't know where Mr. Hotel Manager is.' Then he called a bright young man, who looked at me and said, 'I'm sorry you've been delayed but the manager left a few minutes ago for a business conference. He said he would be back by 3 P.M. If you want to wait, you may have a seat in the lobby, or I can take you to our private waiting room, or you may go shopping for a while.'

"I was touched by the young man's courteous spirit and believed he was telling the truth. Smiling, I said to him, 'Thank you very much for your suggestions. I think I'll shop a while.' . . . By the way, I had never been in that hotel before—its elegance somewhat overwhelms the novice. I went in with dignity and a degree of confidence; I left with both my dignity and my confidence intact."

I asked her two questions:

"Were you really frightened at any time?"

"No."

"Were you at the boiling point enough to lose your temper?"

"No . . . to be honest, almost at the bank, but I really kept cool, honest!"

"You're on your way toward big game. . . . The way you responded in those three situations, you will respond in the close relations which make or break you . . . *healthy assertiveness* is the password. Within the next two or three weeks, there will be many times when you otherwise would permit people to put you down, to walk all over you—your daughter, your mother, your husband, your superior on the job. Each time you will respond strongly and affirmatively. You will face each situation as it comes."

Marilyn said slowly, but with determination, "You know, I believe I can do it."

Before *one* week had passed, Marilyn had to confront each of the persons in the constellation of her important relations: When her daughter demanded a new gown with an outrageous price, Marilyn said in a firm but strong voice, "I realize how important graduation is, but four years of high school should have taught you something about fiscal responsibility within the family. . . . You can get a new dress for half the money; the balance will go toward your college tuition next year."

The daughter was shocked to hear her mother make a flat refusal of her demand. She started to quarrel with her. Marilyn replied, "There's been a disagreement, there will be *no* argument, the case of the two-hundred-dollar gown is settled."

Marilyn's mother had to be dealt with and the disagreement concerned the gown. Mother insisted that the gown should be purchased, graduation is just once, etc., etc. "Mother, it will be to the advantage of all of us if you keep your mouth shut and remain out of this little dispute." Mother was stunned by the new Marilyn.

Husband was more difficult. His unemployment check had not arrived that week. As usual, he demanded money from Marilyn. "I know how much you make at that goddam magazine. . . . You can let me have at least a hundred dollars and never miss it."

She responded: "The days when you can tell me what I must do with my money are over. . . . I've tried to be fair with you, but you will bleed me no longer."

"Then I'm leaving . . . getting out of this crummy place." This was the threat that always melted Marilyn . . . she would melt.

"If that's the way you feel, the sooner you leave, the better it will be for all of us. . . . Your presence in recent months and years has caused nothing but tension. Make up your mind before I get home tonight." She left him with his mouth hanging open.

Then came Mr. Superior. He rushed madly into Marilyn's office waving a copy of an article he had written for the great weekly news magazine. "Why in hell did you let this pass in this shape? . . . You—"

Marilyn rose from her chair, kept her voice low but steady, and said, "I've taken all the crap from you that I am going to take. You wrote the article; you gave it to me to read. However, until this day, you've never given me permission to change or delete one sentence."

He started to interrupt her.

Marilyn continued, "Wait until I am finished. . . . You live and thrive on chaos, and I'm sick of it. Today I shall offer my resignation to Mr. Upper Superior or I shall ask for a transfer within the firm, and I will make my reasons known."

He was confounded but managed to say, "Go ahead . . . resign, anything, just so you get the hell out of here."

Marilyn knew who she was, knew what her background and experience had to offer . . . she could have landed another position with the magazine's chief competitor within days. She began methodically to clear her desk. Within the hour Mr. Superior was in her office. "Marilyn, I apologize. . . . Please don't leave. . . . I know the rest of the office force holds me in contempt . . . if you resign or ask for a transfer, it will be the end of me here. . . . Please, I've a wife, two kids, and a mother-in-law to look after."

As Marilyn completed the reconstruction of these events, especially the one with her superior, a faint smile played around her lips and shone in her eyes. "I feel sorry for the miserable jackass. . . . He's washed up. At fifty he's an old and perhaps a dying man." Then, with too much hardness in her voice, but still smiling to herself, she said, "I'll have his job within two years."

Marilyn was a new person, her life style was completely transformed, and of all this I approved, but I hope that the hypnotic sessions will not take her too far in the other direction!

VI

Asthma—It Just Went Away

There are certain people with whom more time must be spent in a preliminary session than others.

Currently I am working with several psychiatrists and analysts. The reasons for their coming to me are varied. One thing they have in common: during their years of formal education they were never introduced to the subject of hypnosis. Now that hypnosis is on the rise in many parts of the world, these men want to find out, on a personal basis, what it's all about. This tool, used professionally, might conceivably be an aid in their therapeutic work.

Due to their background it was not necessary to spend as much time in a preliminary session as I did with Joan, a thirty-one-year-old high-school teacher in New York. Joan's family physician suggested she try hypnosis. She was suffering from a severe case of asthma, but the physician was wise enough to distinguish between a condition that was psychosomatic and one that was physiological—an end result of emotional condition rather than one which grew out of biological disturbance.

Joan's discomfort was aggravated by her cat, whom she adored. She lived in Manhattan, her family on Long Island. Recently she took the cat to the Long Island home and left it with her parents. So long as she was away from the cat, no asthma; at home for a weekend, out came the oral inhalator with Isuprel or Primatene. She suffered all the symptoms. Her physician suspected that a clue to her trouble, more emotional than physical, lay in Joan's statement that her cat was the one and only cat which precipitated asthmatic attacks. She came to my office; a more tense, fearful person I have rarely seen. Of hypnosis she knew nothing except what she had seen on stage or television where people were made to do ridiculous things. So her first visit (more than an hour) had to be spent attempting to dispel her fears and misconceptions, rather than engaging in a hypnotic session. Every old wives' tale, every incredible myth concerning hypnosis, Joan clung to. But what was she to do? She suffered severe asthmatic attacks, and her physician had recommended she try hypnosis. She was willing to follow her doctor's recommendation.

The myths concerning hypnosis are well known to every person in this field, and in one way or another, or to a lesser degree than another, the myths must be dealt with. Joan's list of worries and the answers to them went something like the following:

1. *Will I be unconscious and "black out"?* Under hypnosis one is aware of what is said and done. True, there is time distortion, as well as an altered state of consciousness. The latter is contested by some, but in the laboratory, working with the electroencephalogram, I have proved to my own satisfaction, if not to others, that hypnosis *is* an altered state of the mind. But this state is neither bad nor dangerous. It simply means that sounds and experiences are usually amplified, played out on a larger screen. Of course, if one is extremely tired he may drop off into delta sleep—restorative sleep. The operator may let the subject sleep for a couple of minutes, then snap his fingers and bring him out of the sleep state and continue the hypnotic process.

2. *If the hypnotist puts me in a trance, has a heart attack and dies while I am under, what happens to me?* I assured Joan that she would move into a state of sleep. This would last about five or ten minutes. I laughed and said, "Hopefully, my body would have been removed before you awakened."

3. *Can I be made to perform acts which are unacceptable to me?* It has been demonstrated that such is not the case. The hypnotic state will be broken immediately if a suggestion is made which the subject considers to be in bad taste, is offensive in any way, or creates greater anxiety. The subject retains his autonomy. He and the person with whom he is working are vibrating together. Each is contributing to a healing situation.

4. *Will I lose my memory or will my memory be weakened?* Just the opposite is true. There is in hypnosis what I call the "psychic

fallout." I have known subjects who are helped by hypnosis for cigarette addiction, etc. Soon after the sessions were over, they noticed
an increase in memory, in both recall and retention. There is often
improvement in the power to concentrate and in the extension of
the interest span. The reason for this "fallout" is simple. Hypnosis
does two things for the individual which are not done by a pill, an
injection, or a knife. At one and the same time it gives him a clearer
mind and a relaxed body. When the physician prescribes a tranquilizer, the patient is tranquilized, mental processes are slowed,
and relaxation of the body is achieved. If he prescribes an "upper,"
the patient usually becomes uptight in more ways than one.

5. *In case my asthma goes away, will I develop another symptom?* "Such as what?" I asked. "Well," she said, "something like
scratching my fingers or picking my nose." I have tried to assure the
reader that this view of "symptom exchange" or "symptom substitute" has largely been discredited. I can think of several rut-ridden
analysts of a certain persuasion who still hold to this view, but these
people have not changed a point or an idea in their psychological
system for more than thirty or forty years. For such healers the
"cause" must be discovered if it takes ten years, or else you get
"symptom substitute."

At this point in our preliminary, get-acquainted session, I could
have begun probing Joan's mind with a multitude of direct and in-
direct questions hoping to discover "why" she became an asthmatic
two years ago. What about her parents? Did they love her or did
she ever feel rejected by them? How did she get along with an older
sister? Did the parents appear to love the sister more than they did
her? What about her work? Perhaps the grueling job of teaching
high school in Manhattan was getting to her. Then I would have
turned to her relationships with friends. Did female friends like her
or did they seem to like her too much? What about men? (Joan was
just getting over a year-long relationship with a married man. She
contributed this bit of information during her second session.) On
and on we could have gone—for months, perhaps years. If during
the sessions she became more enlightened as to the "why," we
would consider that an extra dividend. *But it would not get rid of
the asthma attacks.*

Joan came for her next appointment two days later. This was her *first* hypnotic session. She was tense but determined. I explained to her that all we would do that day would be to attempt to relieve tensions and help her relax as much as possible. The session went well. I followed, with slight variations, the same method of induction previously described, but made no posthypnotic suggestions. She reached a medium-level hypnotic state, which meant she would be easy to work with. Concluding the session, I slowly counted to five, indicating that when she opened her eyes, her mind would be bright and clear and her body beautifully relaxed. She opened her eyes. The tension had left her. Even the features in her face had changed. Joan, who was only thirty-one, had already begun to develop telltale horizontal lines across the forehead and vertical lines up and down the bridge of her nose. Both of these signs disappeared. I knew I was on the right track.

During the second hypnotic session, when we reached the point where posthypnotic suggestions were made, I said, "Joan, the subconscious part of your mind has emerged and gained control over your body, as well as over the conscious part of your mind. The subconscious is your best friend, your friend and ally. It will help you achieve every reasonable and worthy goal you have in life. Your subconscious rejects completely the idea that being with your cat can produce within you asthmatic attacks. When you go to Long Island this weekend, *play with the cat.* If it wants to sleep on the bed with you, that's fine. Let it. You will feel no discomfort. This week you may discard the inhalator."

Joan was to return for a third appointment Monday after a weekend with her cat. Instead she called and said, "It worked . . . it worked! Everybody is surprised, but not I. I don't need another session. From the first talk we had I believed it was going to work, and it did. The attacks have just gone away!"

I haven't seen Joan since that last session. But she calls about every three months to keep me informed. No more asthma and she is neither scratching her fingers nor picking her nose.

On several occasions I have referred to different levels in hypnosis. Explanation of these levels is in order at this point. In 1963, I did intensive research with twelve students, six men and six women, above the freshman class at Bucknell University, where I served as one of the denominational chaplains. Not one of these students ever knew that I was working with any other student. I did not want them to compare notes or playfully conspire against me and the project. I also maintained secrecy because I feel reasonably sure that the administration at Bucknell would not have approved. I was attempting to discover who makes a good subject and who makes a poor subject.

Toward the end of the school year I thought I had made some solid progress. It was beginning to appear that an ultraresponsive subject was rather bright and able to concentrate, had strong imagination and a rapport with the operator, and was eager for the experience. However, I found one subject who fitted none of the descriptions, and he could go into the deepest trance level. And vice versa—there was one student (male) who fitted perfectly the description of the responsive subject, but he was non-hypnotizable, at least he was not hypnotizable by me. Not only was he bright and eager, but he seemed even more than the other students to like me as a person. From the beginning we had excellent rapport. I was baffled by our (mine and his) failure to achieve induction. I saw the subject twice a week for three weeks. Somewhere in his psyche there was a powerful but unconscious resistance to his being hypnotized even though rapport, trust, and motivation had been established. So we do not know who will make a responsive subject until a thorough check and "run-through" has been done. I have heard tales about "stage" hypnotists who can tell within seconds by looking at the pupils of the eyes of a prospective subject, or staring at his hands or feet, whether or not such a subject would be a "good" subject or a "poor" one. I seriously doubt the truth in this. The chances are the entertainer has had some contact with these people prior to the performance.

During this school year at Bucknell, I worked out a system of categorizing subjects. It is my own, but does not seriously differ from that of others in this field, such as R. W. Husband and L. W. Davis. Following are the levels which have meaning for me: 1a–1b; 2a–2b; 3a–3b.

LEVEL ONE—Least Responsive

1a 1a people are on the borderline of being non-hypnotizable. The hypnotic level is something like an IQ level; it may move a little, but not much. If a 1a subject should work with several hypnotists, he may move to 1b level, *but he will not move to the most responsive level, which is 3b.* In the 1a state the one, and perhaps only, characteristic is mild relaxation.

1b Fluttering of eyelids, plus a sense of relaxation and loss of tension. Eyelids may become heavy, but no rigidity in the limbs.

LEVEL TWO—Medium Responsive

2a Extreme heaviness of eyelids, head droops, deep relaxation and loss of tension.

2b Same as 2a, plus limb rigidity, slight numbness in hands, posthypnotic response. (Positive suggestion is given, the subject will carry it out.)

LEVEL THREE—Ultra Responsive

3a Subject can open the eyes and engage in conversation without breaking the trance. Anesthesia and regression (to age five or six).

3b This is the lowest level—the most responsive to the hypnotic process. Characteristics include all of the above, plus complete numbness and the absence of pain. Rigidity of the entire body, dramatic changes in the *five* senses resembling hallucination, especially sight, smell, and taste. Movement into deep sleep. Responsive to suggestions concerning dreams—that is, people who contend that they *never* remember a dream will begin to remember dreams. When a posthypnotic suggestion of a specific dream is given, the subject will have that dream *that night* and he will remember it. Of course, the emphasis on such dreams is characterized by *pleasant suggestions.* This method is useful with people who suffer from certain phobias as well as sexual disabilities.

One would assume that the more responsive the subject, the more effective the results. In most cases this is true, but there are many exceptions. People who are less responsive to the hypnotic process often obtain excellent results.

Percentages of people in the different levels are classified as follows:

10%	non-hypnotizable
25%	1a–1b light–medium responsive
40%	2a–2b medium–heavy responsive
25%	3a–3b heavy responsive

Angie, the second rape victim, was 3b; Marilyn, passive and nonassertive, was 1b and moved to 2b; Joan, psychosomatic asthma, was 2a and moved to 2b.

VII
Students, Professor, and Mind Expansion

1. College Students Learn to Release the Trapdoor

On brief occasions I worked with colleagues on a variety of research problems relating to hypnosis. However, for more than a year I was quietly doing work on my own in the area of memory and mind expansion. I sought out three of my favorite students, whom I shall call Mark, Luke, and John, third-year students in the Divinity School, one of a number of graduate schools at Yale. When I explained to them the type of work we would be engaged in, they jumped at the opportunity to participate. The men varied in temperament as well as scholastic ability; however, all three were graduates of first-rate colleges. Each of them except Mark had hopes of going for the Ph.D. degree upon graduation.

Mark was tall and lean, a former All-American basketball player in college. He was a good student but was not at the top of his class. Required field work found him instructing in athletics at the downtown Y.

Luke's college major had been in drama. He was an esthete, a mild-mannered fellow who reveled in classical music and poetry. Several of his poems had been published by the university press.

John was in many ways the cleverest and most interesting of the three. He graduated Phi Beta Kappa from Princeton, majoring in philosophy. Following college graduation, he took off for Europe and other places unknown on a cargo ship, working as cook and man of all trades. He returned to the States within a year and a half, went to Greenwich Village, and for a brief time became one of that generation's "flower children." Being a natural mimic, he soon was

performing in Village clubs and low-level night spots. One Saturday
night a young woman whom he had met at the club where he was
working invited him to go to church with her the next morning.
"You must be kidding," he said with considerable scorn. She
laughed and said, "Not at all. . . . It's unique."

He was totally committed to non-faith as it applied to religion.
However, by nature he was a curious animal. Though he stayed at
her apartment that night, he did not remember her name. However,
together the next morning they attended the Judson Memorial
Church, where the Rev. Howard Moody is the senior minister and
the Rev. Al Carmines is minister. Howard is a graduate of Yale
Divinity School; Al is a graduate of New York's Union Theological
Seminary. The Judson church has its tradition in Baptist history
and therefore there are no supervising bishops or set liturgies. Each
Baptist church retains its autonomy. John was astounded at the
improvisation in the service, the youthful congregation, the sense of
community, and the unique liturgical service conducted by the two
ministers. Al Carmines was then beginning a career which, according to critic Clive Barnes, has since taken him to the top in New
York's musical circles. After fifteen years Moody and Carmines are
still together, offering people, young and old, unique experiences in
the realm of religion; these include art, music, poetry, politics,
drama, serious study, spontaneous worship, and community concern. John was so impressed that he applied the next year for
admission as a student in the Yale Divinity School. He married the
young lady he met in the Village, the one who took him to church.
His parents had died before he was ten years old and left him a
small fortune in trust. He had little background in religion except
what he experienced at Judson. He was now considered the
number-one student in his senior class. He planned to teach the
philosophy of religion at the college level. John had his heart set on
being accepted in the Ph.D. program at Yale.

As far as I could tell, the three men had fewer problems than
most of us. I chose them because I knew them better than the other
students, and also because I wanted to see if my approach to in-
creasing recall and retention in memory, concentration, and mind
expansion would be as effective with bright students as with slow or
dull ones. In a preliminary session together, prior to induction, I

explained to them the experiment we would attempt in memory. I said, "All of you have had the experience of attempting to recall a name either of a person in your presence or from a book you've read. The name does not come. . . . You try and try, it will not come. Yet you know the person's name as well as your own."

They grinned and nodded. John said, "It happens to me often. I start to introduce this fellow in our class to my wife and I am dumfounded that I can't recall his name." The other two men had similar experiences many times.

I said, "There is a mythical trapdoor lying between your subconscious and your conscious; the chances are, when you are relaxed or at ease, perhaps listening to music or engaging in a non-exciting conversation with another friend, the lost name will pop into your mind."

They agreed that this was true.

"Now," I said, "you will learn recall and retention by the use of a blackboard." I asked Mark to remain and gave the other two men the time and the day of their appointments. When I was alone with Mark, I said, "Ready for a session?"

He said, "Okay."

Induction was quick and easy with Mark, as it proved to be with the other two subjects. While he was still in the trance I explained to him what I meant by the "blackboard method." "This is recall without effort. In other words, you write on the board in huge numbers and letters. When I bring you out of the trance and ask you to repeat what is written, you will not use the memory, you will simply look at the board and read what is there. Understand?"

"I understand."

"To each of the six sessions I will add numbers, letters, and words and perhaps an alphabet, so that at the end of the sixth and last session you will read back to me a full page or more and you will do this without effort."

Mark said softly, "I don't understand how I am to do this without using my memory."

"You will do it by seeing and reading that which you have written on the board."

"Still don't get it . . . but I'm all for it . . . sounds too good to be true." In the trance his voice was soft but clear.

"Mark, visualize a huge blackboard in front of you. Within the mind you arise, walk to the board, and begin to write numbers which I have recorded in my notebook. Write the numbers with large, wide strokes. Today we shall major only in numbers. . . . here they are: *2-3-9-8-9-6-7-7-6-5-5-4-4-1-3-9-7-5-3-2.* As I repeat aloud these twenty digits, keep the chalk in your hand and write over the numbers one more time, making them sharper and clearer. Within a few minutes I shall ask you to look at the blackboard—you may do so with eyes open or closed, whichever is easier. In a non-forced manner you will read to me what you have written."

I gave the signal, Mark opened his eyes, stretched, and said, "I feel great." There were about two minutes of trivial conversation. Then I said, "Look at the blackboard and read the numbers which you wrote. I will follow along in my notebook. Remember, the trapdoor is wide open, you're relaxed and you will read to me what you see."

With eyes open, he began reading the numbers clearly and accurately with no effort. He exclaimed, "I'll be damned!"

By the second week all three men had reached the "letter" stage. The letters were written on the blackboard just below the numbers.

I was now working with Luke, the esthete. "Write in clear letters the following." Slowly I called the letters: *q-a-z-e-d-c-r-f-v-p-l-m-o-k-n-t-g-b-i-j-b-u-h-w-s-x.*

I brought Luke out of the trance and asked him to read what he saw on the blackboard. He read quickly and easily, then he stumbled on three letters, *v-p-l,* making them read *l-p-v,* but only for a moment. He smiled and said, "Just a minute, I reversed three letters!" He went back and read *v-p-l* and from there on there was no hesitation.

He said, "Let me try it with my eyes closed."

"Surely."

Eyes closed, he read the letters accurately and without the slightest hesitation.

When we arrived at the words, the mythical board was beginning to look like a Chinese crossword puzzle put together by a very strange person. To the two exercises, I added the following words: *amble, beyond, carrier, dance, electric, finger, ginger, hesitancy, in-*

cident, jester, kidney, liberty, malignant, nucleolus, opera, pantheism, quadruple, random, sacred, tiger, unicorn, vein, wallop, xylophone, yacht, zinc.

After he came out of the trance, I asked John to rest for a moment, then said, "Now read the *numbers, letters,* and *words.*" I followed the three different sets in my notebook. He missed no number, no letter, and no word.

John said, "This is more fun than I have had since I came to this place. How do you explain it?"

"I can't say; I'm not sure anyone can. You were doing it the easy way, just looking and reading."

On two or three occasions we reviewed that which was on the blackboard, ending with the twenty-six words.

The last week was an exercise in an alphabet with which they were not familiar. Mark read and spoke French and German. Luke read and spoke French, Spanish, and German. John was fluent in French, German, Italian, Japanese, and Russian. "How about Greek?" I asked each of them. "No Greek, no Hebrew . . . guess we'll get to that later," said John. (These languages were not required at the Divinity School.)

During the last hypnotic session, I gave them the Greek alphabet to write on the board. John knew Russian and there is a similarity between the two alphabets, but not sufficient to be of help to him in our exercise. At this last session I put the three men in a trance at the same time and said to them, "To the numbers, letters, and words you have written on the blackboard, I now want you to write the Greek alphabet. I will speak slowly. Write in large letters: *alpha-beta-gamma-delta-epsilon-zeta-eta-theta-iota-kappa-lambda-mu-nu-xi-omicron-pi-rho-sigma-tau-upsilon-phi-chi-psi-omega.* I shall repeat slowly. Write in large, clear letters. Two of you will be brought out of the trance; wait in the next room. Mark will remain here; Luke and John will leave the room. Mark, relax and keep your eyes closed as I give suggestions to Luke and John."

The suggestions of a clear mind and relaxed body were given. They responded. Luke said, "I can see the blackboard right now, but I wonder if I'll be able to read what I see." John said, "I'm so relaxed, I feel like taking a nap."

"I will be with Mark not more than fifteen minutes; you may

sit on the couch or the sofa-chair in the room next door. I'll call you when your time comes."

"Mark, how're you feeling?"

"Great."

"Ready to read back to me the entire board?"

"Yes, I'm ready."

In order for the reader to see precisely what was involved, I shall give the entire set of numbers, letters, words, and alphabet as they appeared on the mythical blackboard.

Numbers: 2-3-9-8-9-6-7-7-6-5-5-4-4-1-3-9-7-5-3-2

Letters: q-a-z-e-d-c-r-f-v-p-l-m-o-k-n-t-g-b-i-j-b-u-h-w-s-x

Words: amble, beyond, carrier, dance, electric, finger, ginger, hesitancy, incident, jester, kidney, liberty, malignant, nucleolus, opera, pantheism, quadruple, random, sacred, tiger, unicorn, vein, wallop, xylophone, yacht, zinc

Alphabet: alpha-beta-gamma-delta-epsilon-zeta-eta-theta-iota-kappa-lambda-mu-nu-xi-omicron-pi-rho-sigma-tau-upsilon-phi-chi-psi-omega

To Mark, I said, "You have gradually grown more and more relaxed. The blackboard appears before you . . . *numbers, letters, words, alphabet.* What you have written on the board now becomes increasingly clear. Look at the entire board for a few moments. Then read what you see."

Mark, the slowest of the students, began to read. He did not hesitate. He read every number, every letter, every word, and the Greek alphabet without halting once.

I brought him out of the trance and he snapped his fingers and said, "I did it . . . I know I did."

"You certainly did . . . not a miss."

Luke and John came in, each at his turn. Each was put once again into a trance. The same suggestions were given . . . blackboard, clear; numbers, letters, words, and alphabet, bright and sharp. Each subject repeated perfectly.

When I brought them out of the trance, Luke was quiet, but John said, "What's the meaning? What have we done? How will it affect our lives?"

I laughed and said, "Now you become the teacher. Each of you must tell me within the next three months what, if anything, has radically changed in your life. . . . Does the trapdoor between subconscious and conscious open any easier? Can you write names, places, dates, etc., on the blackboard and recall with ease? Are your powers of concentration improved?"

Within a few weeks, Mark stopped me on campus. "Good Lord," he said, "the one thing I could not do was to remember names. Now, I just write names on the board and recall them at will."

Luke's contribution: "You know how I love poetry. For some mysterious reason I have had difficulty committing to memory certain choice passages which have meant a great deal to my life. Now I write them on the board and there they are!"

I saw John and his lovely wife in a restaurant near New Haven. He came over to the table and said, "Professor Myers is letting me in his Greek class. It is an advanced class, but since I know languages pretty well, it should be a breeze." Then he laughed and said, "Especially since I have the blackboard to work with."

Mark decided to go into the parish ministry once he received his degree in the spring; Luke did not make the Yale School of Graduate Studies but was accepted by another ranking university. John was accepted, one of four students out of a hundred in the Divinity School, for Yale's Ph.D. program.

Previously, at the University of North Carolina, I had collaborated with a number of students on this type of research, but not quite so intensively. In recent years, I have worked successfully with dozens of people who are short on memory and concentration, using the "blackboard method."

2. The Professor—Publish or Perish

The man sitting before me was a contradiction in terms. He was Dr. Isaac R., assistant professor of English literature at Yale College. He began as instructor, completed his Ph.D., and was promoted to assistant professor, which meant that he, at the age of thirty-six, had been a member of the faculty of this university for about eight or nine years, the only full-time position he had ever held. It was predicted by his colleagues that Isaac would soar to academic heights and become one of the nation's authorities in his chosen field. However, for months his work was downhill. He found himself under the edict of "publish or perish." By publish, the administration and senior faculty meant not just an article or two, but an acceptable scholarly book.

Isaac came to my office on the first floor of Yale's Divinity School and tried to tell me how he felt about himself, his work, and his future. He had made a dozen starts at "the" book and tried to outline it; he did more research, but could not sit down at the typewriter and sweat it out. He said, "I'm afraid it will not be up to standard; the faculty will sneer at my efforts; academic critics will tear me apart."

"All you need is something that can move you to that typewriter."

He continued, "Maybe I've had it. I peaked too soon. I can't live up to the expectations of either friends or family. The book cannot be finished; I will not receive tenure, and I'll be out looking for another job." Then he made a statement full of emotion, but I was sure it was for the moment and not a true evaluation of his work. With clenched fist he said, "I hate this goddamn teaching job more than anything else. Maybe it will be good for me to get out of it."

He paused for a long time. I waited. At last he asked, "Do you think hypnosis can help me out of this blue funk?"

My reply was serious, and Isaac took it so to be. I said, "You have a greater chance of being helped by hypnosis *if you believe you can be helped.*"

I knew that the young professor shared not only resistance to, but contempt for, this area of work to which I have been committed for so long. The antagonistic attitudes of academic as well as church communities toward hypnosis have been so strong that I have had to keep a sense of humor about it and in early years referred to myself as a "closet hypnotist." If Isaac could, to a degree, overcome his resistance to hypnosis, I felt he could be helped. This I bluntly conveyed to him.

He was tight, tense, insecure, and afraid. His academic life, prior to Yale, was that of the overachiever; now he was the underachiever. He graduated summa cum laude from a little-known college. His graduate work was on a high level but it also was done at a university not considered strong in liberal arts. So when he arrived at Yale, feeling sure he would be promoted "up the ladder," he extended himself. His lectures were prepared with care, his students found him a hard master but fair. However, there were times when he could not accept working in such a rarefied academic atmosphere, not to mention rubbing shoulders every day with some of the greatest scholars in the world. So he pushed himself to the limit to make good. One day the Dean asked him to come by his office. He was frightened even though it was a friendly conversation. The Dean said, "Your work has been carefully watched the past several years. We like what we see. However, your tenure as assistant professor is either renewed or terminated in May—eighteen months from now."

Isaac swallowed hard and said, "Yes, sir, I know."

"You, of course, also know our policy. . . . By that time you must write and have published by an acceptable publishing company a work which will satisfy the Committee on Promotions as well as the senior faculty." The Dean paused and said, "Have you as yet put anything on paper?"

"Frankly, no; I've started a dozen times. Writing does not come easily, but I like my work here, and you can rest assured that I'll have a creditable work done by next May."

"We admire you and your work in the classroom. I hope to see the results of your labors by that time. . . . By the way, talk to one or more of your friends on the faculty who by experience know what it is to write that first book. You'll find them encouraging and also able to make helpful suggestions."

"I shall waste no time in doing that. . . . Thank you very much."

The conversation ended. Isaac sought out several friends, all of whom assured him he would have no trouble. But six months went by and he still had not written anything that he would let a friend read. A colleague suggested that he come and talk to me. "What does he do?" Isaac said. "Hypnosis is his major interest, but he teaches pastoral psychology and kindred subjects in the Divinity School."

Isaac was depressed that one of his best friends had no better suggestion than to send him to a hypnotist! However, in desperation he finally made it to my office. During that first visit he was nervous and inquisitive. "I know nothing about hypnosis . . . read a little about Mesmer and Puységur, whose antics appeared to me to be pathological."

"True, they were eccentric men, but when you pioneer in anything, you're likely to make a fool of yourself in more ways than one. Are you ready for a hypnotic session?"

"Yes, I've wasted too much time already."

The procedure I used with Isaac is the simplest known in the field of hypnosis. He had to achieve muscular relaxation, experience loss of emotional tension, and something positive had to happen which would restore confidence in himself as a human being, a real person, and in himself as a professor and scholar. He was reasonably responsive to hypnotic induction. The first four times he came to the office, I did nothing but offer suggestions of relaxation, loss of tension, and gaining confidence.

At the fifth session I made my first move in the direction of a specific posthypnotic suggestion: "You will sort out the research material you have collected, then you will think through the material until you have a central theme around which the book will develop. Then you will write out a table of contents. . . . This will not be firm and final, but it will serve as a guide. Finally, when you come in next time, bring a three-page synopsis of the work you intend to do."

The session was soon over. Isaac said as he left, "Can't wait to get to my office; I'll have that synopsis."

The sixth time he came in he was excited. "Look what I've done."

He had piles and piles of research material, now carefully catalogued and filed in a variety of folders. He explained his theme, which centered on "Genius and Madness in Men of Letters"— confining himself to England's seventeenth, eighteenth, and nineteenth centuries. The table of contents showed a remarkable degree of natural development and the synopsis was simple, direct, and explanatory.

I looked over the material and congratulated him. Then I laughed and said, "Now all you must do is grind out three hundred pages . . . *and you will do that.*"

Isaac said, "Not since completing my graduate work have I felt so confident."

Sessions seven and eight, I requested that he bring in the first draft of chapters one and two, about forty typewritten pages.

At the conclusion of each of these sessions I said, "You will now find it as hard to stay away from the typewriter as you found it easy to run from it a month ago. Not only so, but there will be a sense of excitement, joy, and exhilaration as you realize you are doing not a scissors-and-paste job but a real work of creativity. The exhilaration will be akin to that of an excellent actor as he goes on stage to perform in a work which challenges him. You will be challenged by the work you have started and you will meet that challenge."

Isaac completed his work in March! Two months ahead of schedule. We had broken through his anxiety, his listlessness, his procrastination, his insecurity. The senior faculty praised his manuscript, which was immediately accepted by a New York publisher.

During the month we worked together there was only one period when I felt Isaac was losing ground. Somewhere along the fourth or fifth session he came into my office tense and worried.

Bypassing shop talk, I asked, "What's the trouble today?"

He said, "It's difficult to talk about."

"Perhaps another time."

"Oh, no, I want to talk about it now."

"Fire away."

"I lay awake most of the night thinking . . . just thinking. Do you believe there would be enough opposition on the Committee to force me out even if I write a respectable book?"

"Why would you think such an impossibility?"

By now we were on a first-name basis. "Wesley, as you well know, I am a Jew. . . . Being a Jew has been a problem for me in more places than you could dream of . . . housing in the New Haven area, for instance. I just thought that since there are so few Jews on the faculty, they might turn me down if full tenure were involved."

I looked at him with disbelief. "If you think there is a quota system for Jews on the Yale faculty, you have a misunderstanding of what this university is about. Have you ever felt discriminated against, or pushed aside, because you were a Jew?"

"Only slightly have I ever felt it among faculty members. Students are another breed; at times there is open hostility toward me for no other reason than my being a Jew."

I laughed and said, "If we want to trade bits of paranoia, let me tell you: there are twenty-eight million Baptists in this country and six million Jews. I'm a Baptist. There are fewer Baptists on the university faculty than Jews and fewer Baptist students than Jewish students. I know firsthand the type of brush-off you have felt. To people who should know better, there is nothing stranger or even more obnoxious than a Baptist!"

At this Isaac laughed. "You're right. When I heard that my friend was recommending me to a hypnotist who was a Baptist, I instinctively hesitated."

"You see then what I mean. . . . Isaac, you're a good teacher, of that I'm sure. Write a respectable book before next May, and I'll bet you a trip to Israel that you will be promoted with all the fringe benefits."

From that point on nothing could stop him.

As a result of my encounter with Isaac, he and I became good friends. We enjoyed lunch together about once a week, and also played squash in the gym when time would permit. Due to his firsthand experience, Isaac became fascinated with hypnosis and also with his total ignorance of it. To the latter point, I said he should not feel ashamed of his lack of knowledge in this field; there are scores of physicians, psychiatrists, and psychologists who are ignorant of this subject which is directly related to their field of study and work.

Isaac on his own initiative had begun to read, not so much in the area of techniques of hypnosis but in the history and theories of it. One day at lunch he said, "In the few books I have thus far read, I notice that authorities in hypnosis have a difficult time defining just what hypnosis is."

I laughed and said, "It's non-definable—hypnosis is non-rational and primal. It's as difficult to define as electricity."

Seriously, he said, "What is *your* theory? Is the base from which you operate in hypnosis religious or non-religious?"

"It is religious, a healing power for body and spirit. . . . Concerning my own theory, this I will do: next week when we get together, I will give you a succinct view of the various theories of hypnosis and then an interpretation of my own."

"You mean you'll take the time to write it out for me!"

"Sure . . . it will be good discipline for me."

Next week I handed Isaac a statement of various theories of hypnosis, including the one I hold. I explained to him that having my own view did not mean that I reject all other views. There's some truth in most of them.

We ate a quick lunch. He remarked as we left the coffee shop, "I can't wait to get back to the office to read this."

The sheet I gave to Isaac that day contained the following information concerning "theories" which certain readers may find helpful.

Conditioning. Pavlov, the famous Russian neurophysiologist, based his approach to human behavior on the conditioned reflex. Of course, you know about the famous dog and the famous bell. Every time the dog was fed, a bell would ring. Within a short period of time the hungry dog associated eating food with the ringing of the bell. Soon the bell would ring but there would be no food; the dog would salivate as quickly as he heard the bell, even though there was no food. Pavlov attempted to demonstrate that people in particular, and society in general, can be conditioned in precisely the same way. People can be conditioned to follow rules or to break rules, they can be conditioned to be nonviolent or to be violent. In the hypnotic trance, one may be conditioned by repeated suggestions to a certain form of behavior. It is relatively easy to do this, if the suggestions are *positive* and *creative*. It is virtually impossible under hypnosis to condition a person in a destructive way. It is easier to condition a person in destructive ways while his mind is conscious and active than it is under hypnosis when the subconscious emerges and takes control. This is probably true because when one is in a trance anxiety may be an ally—nothing will break the hypnotic state quicker than the sudden pulse of anxiety.

Suggestion. This is the theory that insists there is no such thing as hypnosis, and if there were, it would not be necessary to put a person in a trance to secure the type of results which hypnosis is supposed to produce. In other words, if the subject has complete faith in what is going on and the operator has complete confidence in himself, anything that can be produced under hypnosis can be produced simply by repeated suggestions.

Sleep. The word "hypnosis" is from the Greek word *hypnos,* meaning sleep, and is an unfortunate and inaccurate description of hypnosis. If hypnosis is anything in its own right, it is not sleep. And the compromise theory of hypnosis being a halfway station between wakefulness and sleep is just as inaccurate. Hypnosis is a separate and distinct modality unto itself. It may have fathered similar activity, but that does not mean that it has lost its own identity.

The Chess Theory. This theory says that hypnosis is the mover of men who are stopped dead center. In mental institutions and analysts' offices innumerable people seek the kind of help that will enable them to get going—doing something, doing anything. Often psychotherapy is all the individual needs, but there are others who respond neither to psychotherapy nor to chemotherapy. In certain instances a subject, in a state of lethargy, will respond to the hypnotic process. He may, of course, need further therapy, but at least there was something which "got him moving."

The Locked-Vault Theory. Here is an enormous vault which represents the subject's complex mental apparatus. Inside the vault are thousands upon thousands of small, locked boxes. Some have grown crusty with age, not having been opened for years upon years. Hypnosis is the power which not only unlocks the huge vault, but also may open one by one each of the smaller boxes, bringing forth treasures both old and new.

The Universal Mind and the Subconscious Mind. This is the theory which makes more sense to me than any thus far advanced. It gives me a philosophical and religious base from which to work. Though I do not hold C. G. Jung responsible for what I contend to be the most meaningful theory concerning the mystery of hypnosis, I am indebted to him. It was Jung who helped some of us believe in the universal mind, that collective mind which works for man's good. When the subconscious part of man's mind emerges, it rises to be met by the universal mind of which it is a part.

In the hypnotic process, when one is without doubt in a hypnotic trance, there is a specific time in the person's psyche when the miracle occurs. The miracle is the moment when the *subconscious* takes charge. It takes precedence over the body, over the conscious part of the mind as well as the five senses. In one respect Freud was right about the subconscious. It may well be the "id"—that part of the personality into which we cram all manner of wicked thoughts and memories. Conflicts rage *within* the "id" because they are in opposition with both the distant and the immediate environment, including people who constitute members of the family. However, the subconscious may be the dynamo, the powerhouse that motivates and energizes the personality. When it is released in destructive directions it triggers negative emotions in such a way that a hole can be bored in the stomach; the voice, through hysteria, disappears; non-diagnosable pains occur; etc. However, the subconscious is so powerful that, used *constructively* and *creatively,* it assists a distraught subject to fulfill himself.

When a subject experiences the power of the subconscious he becomes a person who is on top of his problems; his problems are not on top of him. He achieves an upbeat attitude toward life. He does not become more dependent; the autonomous self is strengthened. Hypnosis is the art of tapping that substance (*the universal mind*) which, like glue, holds the universe together. Hypnosis is not rational; neither is it irrational. It is primal and non-rational; it provides an experience into which one may enter in confidence and without intellectualizing (endlessly) and from which one takes as much of the substance into himself as possible.

The statement I gave Isaac ended with these words:

A successful hypnotic experience means exchanging an unwholesome life style for a wholesome one. It means overcoming damaging habits and breaking destructive addictions, it means relieving tension and achieving a meaningful type of serenity, it deals constructively with deep-seated fears, it means the improvement of memory and calling forth the powers of concentration, it brings to the surface buried skills and talents. It forces initiative where there has been listlessness, it assists one to move toward the reasonable and worthy goals he has in life.

There were not many members of the faculty of the Divinity School with whom I could discuss the various aspects of hypnosis. Therefore, I cherished Isaac's friendship for more reasons than one.

VIII

The Insomniac Learns to Sleep

Lines laced his face, fear showed in his eyes, and his voice trembled. "I tried to kill myself because I have grown to hate the night. For years night after night I have lain awake thinking, thinking, thinking; then fighting, fighting, fighting. Why did I do it?"

I said, "At this point I am not interested in attempting to discover why you slashed your wrists, I am more interested in helping you with your insomnia."

Peter, age fifty-four, had been president of a large advertising firm in New York. He retired at age fifty-two, after having been with the same firm for thirty years. When I first met him five years ago, he was handsome, bright, and looked ten or fifteen years younger than his age. His inability to sleep had done him in. He was rapidly on his way toward becoming a disabled old man long before his time.

Peter had read a number of books on insomnia. He already knew what has become obvious; namely, that there are many distinctive traits involving one's pattern of sleep. Some people require less sleep than others; five hours of restorative sleep without drugs or alcohol are more satisfying than nine hours with drugs or alcohol.

Peter knew about the REM (rapid eye movement) period, which indicates the dreaming portion of sleep. It is in the dream period when one's subconscious mind attempts to deal with anger, frustration, insecurity, and hostility. He accepted the latter view rather than attaching any precognitive interpretation to his dreams— precognitive meaning that one dreams, for instance, of his mother's death during the night and she dies the next day. I felt that he brushed off certain possible precognitive factors in the dream life but did not argue with him about this.

Peter did not know that a hard-core insomniac may be suffering from psychological trauma which produces a type of hysteria resembling that of the person who under great stress loses the use of the voice or becomes blind or a limb is paralyzed. When younger, he believed that a strong sexual orgasm produced natural sleep; he no longer believed that it did. "My wife is very patient," he said. "She and I still sleep in the same room and the same bed . . . king size. The frequency of sex has nothing to do with how I sleep . . . sometimes I get a little drowsy, but just as often I become more awake."

If I were the probing kind, I would have guessed that Peter's early retirement from a thriving, hectic, challenging position may have started him on the path to drugs or to drinking too much alcohol. However, I was more interested in helping him break the insomnia syndrome than spending months trying to discover the many—not one or two—reasons why he could not secure for himself restorative sleep. He was now off sleeping pills and his use of liquor had been reduced to minor proportions, but his insomnia was worse.

I said, "You seem to have read a great deal about sleep and insomnia. What have you read? What do you know about hypnosis?"

"Absolutely nothing. . . . My secretary of several years ago, a two-pack-a-day smoker, came to you for assistance. Since the second session, she has not smoked one cigarette. I thought you may have worked with people with this damnable problem of insomnia."

"I have had some success and some failure." Actually the insomniac is as difficult to work with successfully as is the alcoholic or stutterer.

Several years ago a large distributing company asked me to write a script and cut a tape—the tape was called *Sleep without Alcohol or Drugs*. My conclusions about the tape are not all in; however, I do believe now that the tape is effective only with the mild type of insomniac, not with as serious a one as Peter. However, during our first session I asked him if he would like to try the tape then and there. He was eager to do so. Deviating from the sitting position, I asked him to stretch out on the couch, close his eyes, and listen as peacefully as possible to the entire tape, thirty minutes. As the tape concluded its full run, Peter opened his eyes, sat up, and said, "I feel somewhat rested, but I never approached sleep . . . even the slightest."

I had used the tape in this way scores of times and with varying degrees of success. The mild insomniac moves from relaxation to loss of tension, to a trancelike condition, to deep restorative sleep. Not so with Peter. I said, "Obviously the tape has little effect on you. Would you like to come in for several additional sessions? You will be put into a trance, and I shall give you a variety of post-hypnotic suggestions."

Peter said, "I will gladly come in for as long as you say. . . . I'll do anything. . . . When can I see you again?"

I looked at my calendar. "Friday at four."

We shook hands and I said, "While we are working, do not read anything about hypnosis."

"Reason?"

"There are times when a little reading is good; there are other times when it retards the remedy."

Friday at four, Peter came in looking as he did the first time I saw him—face lined, fear in his eyes, voice trembling.

"Get any sleep last night?"

"Thirty minutes at a time . . . eleven till five . . . guess about three or four hours."

I explained that during the trance I would ask him to talk to me, perhaps answer several questions. He would do so in a clear, controlled voice.

The induction went well. We reached the "breathing of sleep" period; he was in a deep hypnotic state. The time had come for the first posthypnotic suggestion. "Peter, in these hypnotic sessions we must break the insomniac syndrome. In my judgment you developed this pattern by learning it and becoming habituated to it. You must unlearn it, and the pattern of habit must be broken. Do you hear me and do you understand me?"

"Yes, I hear you . . . not sure I understand fully." His voice was strong and clear.

"I mean, in order to break your present pattern, we must develop another. The one we will work on first will be to help you become a day sleeper instead of a night sleeper. Do you understand now?"

"I think so."

"Tonight, you will stay up all night as if you had the late shift on the police force. Do not take your clothes off. Get ready for bed about nine o'clock in the morning and sleep as long as possible."

Peter smiled in the trance. "My wife will think I'm crazy for sure."

"You said she was quite tolerant."

"Really, she is; she'll do anything if it helps. How long do I keep this up?"

"For seven nights, stay up all night, retiring each morning about nine o'clock."

"I'll do it," he said firmly.

He came out of the trance and said, "My God, I am relaxed. . . . First time I've felt at ease in a long time."

"While you were in the trance, was there a time when you went into sleep, when you could not hear my voice?"

"Briefly, once or twice."

"Can you recall my posthypnotic suggestion?"

He thought for a moment and said, "Yes . . . yes, I'm to break the present pattern by developing a new one: sleep daytime instead of night."

"Correct . . . and you will begin tonight."

One week later, Peter came in. He looked rested, less harassed.

"How'd it go?" I asked.

"It worked." Then he laughed and said, "But it's killing my wife."

"Give me a rundown on the week."

Peter described in detail how his pattern, sleep from eleven o'clock at night to seven o'clock in the morning, was broken. "The first night I did as you suggested, I stayed up all night . . . no booze. Got into bed, slept soundly until two in the afternoon. Sleep was unbroken and I felt great."

"Go on."

"The next night, it was a little harder to stay awake, but I made it . . . slept about seven daylight hours, uninterrupted. So it has gone each day and night."

"Ready for another session?"

"Sure. . . . What will it be this time?"

"Have you ever been athletic . . . swim or golf, etc.?"

"You bet. . . . I was a champion hundred-yard swimmer in college. Played tennis and golf."

"Have you done anything lately?"

"Nine holes of golf, once a week."

"What does your doctor say about your condition . . . especially your heart?"

"He was surprised as hell when they took me to the hospital with my wrists slashed. . . . I had just been to him for a thorough checkup. He gave me a good one. He's an excellent man. At the time, he prescribed more sleeping pills and said, 'I really don't know why you need these. You are as healthy as a horse, especially the old ticker. Many a man of forty wishes he had a heart as strong as yours.' My blood pressure was excellent, cholesterol perfect."

"All right, Peter, get ready . . . close your eyes for a few moments, take five nice deep breaths, notice as you let the breath out each time that your body will become increasingly relaxed. Up, one . . . hold for a second; down slowly; up, two . . . hold, down slowly, relaxing all the way; up, three, hold . . . down slowly; up four, hold, down slowly; now for the deepest, up, up, hold for a second, down and relax. . . ."

By this time Peter was beginning the hypnotic trance. I continued, "The pattern must be changed again. Stay up all night tonight, to bed about seven in the morning, arise at one in the afternoon. Go to the golf course and play twenty-seven holes of golf."

"Twenty-seven?"

"Yes, twenty-seven. Following golf, take a hot shower, eat a satisfying meal . . . no liquor. As soon as you feel sleep approaching, get ready for bed—no matter the time of night. Set the alarm one hour from the time you get in bed. When the alarm goes off, get up, set it to ring two hours later, go back to bed, you will immediately fall asleep. When the alarm goes off a second time, get up, turn it off, but do not reset it. Again, you will go back to bed and this time sleep until you are refreshed. Do you understand?"

"I understand. Is that all?"

"No, the procedure of twenty-seven holes of golf will be repeated three days straight going—if weather permits. The procedure of setting the alarm and resetting it as outlined will continue."

"Is that all?"

"Not quite. . . . During the following two days, in the late afternoon, play tennis until you're tired. Go through the same procedure . . . hot shower, good evening meal, get ready for bed, set the alarm as before."

"Is that all?"

"Not quite. . . . The last day before coming in, go to the gym and swim . . . swim until you're tired. Follow the same pattern, then I shall see you one week from today."

I continued, "When I count to five you may open your eyes. You will eagerly look forward to the assignments given you, and this week you will sleep as directed."

Peter came in for the third session. We had been working together for three weeks. Bags under his eyes had almost cleared up, the lines in his face were less prominent, fear in the eyes was gone, and his voice was strong and steady. As he sat down he looked at me and laughed and asked, "What in the hell are you doing to me? Am I a rabbit or a little white mouse? Are you doing some kind of research or experimentation?"

I smiled and said, "No, Peter, I'm not doing research and I'm not experimenting. . . . I'm simply trying to help you conquer one of the most difficult malfunctions in life."

"How did you get so deep into this subject?"

"It's not a topic I usually talk about, but for ten years I suffered the agonies of hell with sleeplessness similar to yours. Mine began with the use of sleeping pills, which I needed following a long period of hospitalization. Prior to entering the hospital for surgery, I was a 'good' sleeper. Six or seven hours were all I needed. I would awaken every morning at six-thirty or seven feeling in great shape . . . usually to the disgust of my family—whistling and singing and ready for the day. I allowed myself to get hooked on sleeping pills, and I cannot blame the physician. The pressure I applied to him was: 'I can't do my daily work without the pills.' And he would give them to me."

"You had it that bad?"

" 'Bad' is the word. . . . I had access to the material of the sleep-and-dream programs at Yale and studied them carefully. I went to Russia not simply to learn their approach to hypnosis and parapsychology but to learn about their program of electrosleep."

"Seems that I have heard about it but do not know what it is."

"It is the induction of sleep by the use of a machine called the Electrosom. It stimulates the lower regions of the brain. Electrodes are placed on the head, usually above both temples and the forehead. Mild impulses are then sent to the 'sleep' area of the brain.

"These then produce a relaxing sensation which leads directly into conventional sleep. Some people sleep a few hours and are rested; some must sleep longer to achieve the same rest. At any rate, Russia has about 275 of these clinics and they appear to be getting positive results."

"Why don't we have such machines in this country?"

"For the reason that our scientists have tried similar but not the same machines and the results have not been good."

"Did you try electrosleep in Russia?"

"No, one of my closest friends was a specialist in hypnosis in Chapel Hill, North Carolina. I went to see him hoping that a hypnotic program would assist me. Self-induction completely failed with my type of insomnia."

"What method did he use?"

"Peter, he used the same system I have used with you. I had been practicing hypnosis for about fifteen years at the time, but I knew little about helping people with this sickness. . . . I call it sickness because I believe that's what it is. I thought my friend had flipped out, but, like you, I was desperate. I did not let him know my reservation but immediately started his program, using my full summer vacation."

"What was his explanation of why this sort of program works when typical suggestions of relaxation, loss of tension, etc., do not?"

"Dr. Forrester explained that no one knows for sure why we have sleep patterns common to our own personality—it may be heredity or it may be environment, it may be habituation—*we are creatures of habit*. He felt that sleep patterns were the result of conditioning over a period of years. The individual feels that he must go to bed at a certain hour and wake up at a certain time. Some people cannot sleep on a bed other than their own, nor can they sleep on any side of the bed other than the one they are accustomed to. Some must sleep with bedclothes over them even in summer, while others sleep in the raw in cold weather. The variety of individual habits and eccentricities concerning sleep are endless. Dr. Forrester insisted that one is not freed from the chains of sleep habits until he overcomes these traits so that he can sleep anywhere, any time, and under any conditions."

Peter laughed and said, "After these two weeks, I think I'm getting there fast. . . . Good God, I can't believe I set the alarm twice each night for a week and then went back to sleep! For a guy who had to use his favorite pillow as a security blanket, I think I've made progress."

"Certainly you've made progress, but there're still several weeks to go. Dr. Forrester said that the real test was breaking the time barrier. By that he meant flying from one time zone to another and returning while your body attempts to adjust. It was his view that the 'time lag' is a matter of habit and can be changed or eliminated; one can adjust to it."

"You mean I must fly to Europe and come back the next day?"

"Something like that."

"May the Mrs. accompany me?"

"Not this time . . . go it alone. Besides, it's only fair to give her some rest!"

"I agree. . . . What's the deal and where do I go?"

"Fly from New York to Rome or Madrid. Take your choice . . . spend two nights in either place. Catch an early plane the third morning for San Francisco. Spend two nights in that lovely city."

"Did you do all this flying?"

"No. I didn't have the cash, but you have. Dr. Forrester insisted that this was a necessary part of the treatment. If I had had the money I believe I would have recovered sooner."

"I'm more than willing . . ."

"From San Francisco, take a nonstop to Tokyo, remain *three* nights, and return nonstop to San Francisco. Stay one night in San Francisco, return nonstop to New York the next day."

"What then?"

"Come to see me two days after your return. Take notes on each trip . . . describe your feelings—the ease or difficulty in which you sleep, reactions to time lag and responses to this amount of plane travel, etc., etc."

"Do we have a hypnotic session today?"

"Yes, we do. . . . The posthypnotic suggestions will deal primarily with being able to adjust perfectly to the time lag."

The hypnotic session began and I was again surprised at the ease with which Peter went into a deep-level trance. He was truly a responsive subject.

When he reached the deepest level, I said, "You tell me you've never been afraid to travel by plane . . . it was boring and tiring."

Peter said, "Yes, that's right."

I continued, "You will fly from New York to Rome or Madrid . . . then to San Francisco, from San Francisco to Tokyo, from Tokyo back to San Francisco, then to New York. . . . Peter, do you know how many days this exercise will take?"

"No, but as you outlined it, it must be about twenty."

He was still in a deep trance; talking seemed to deepen his level rather than weakening it. "Not twenty . . . but you're close. It will take sixteen or seventeen days. During that period *time* will have lost all meaning to you. The idea that people *must* sleep at night is nonsense. . . ."

"I agree."

"I have a writer friend who is a night person, another a creative composer of music . . . both of these men are night people . . . they start to work in the quiet of late night and retire about mid-morning."

"I'll be able to do that?"

"Hear me now. . . . These two friends have different sleep patterns than most of us . . . *but they're locked in, the same as you are.* The goal we have set for you is to break all binding habits and be free to sleep when you need it, anywhere, anytime. . . . You will be surprised at the ease with which you make these trips. Take as few clothes as possible, drink little, perhaps a scotch before a meal and a glass of wine with the meal. But here again, do not let this become routine; one day have a drink, the next day or two pass it up. Enjoy the food . . . coach passengers may be given bland food, but in first class you get the best . . . enjoy it. During these traveling days there are three key words, remember them: joy, excitement, euphoria . . . joy, excitement, euphoria . . . these will be the dominant feelings . . . not because you're traveling—you've probably been to these distant places many times."

Peter nodded affirmatively.

"Feelings of joy, excitement, euphoria will be rooted in the certain knowledge that you're overcoming a disease which has haunted you for a number of years and made you a desperate man. Now when you need sleep you will sleep anywhere, anytime, under any conditions. . . . This is a prize more dear than any honor you received in your business and worth more to you than all the money and property you've accumulated."

Peter still in the trance said, "By God, that's right . . . so right."

"Rest and relax for a few moments. Ponder the suggestions I have made, feel the power in the words which are now deep within your mind . . . *joy, excitement, euphoria.*"

I brought him out of the trance. His eyes opened, he began to smile, and finally he said, "I'm making the reservations for the entire trip today."

He left with: "See you two days after I return."

The days went by. Peter called me the day he arrived in New York. "Never felt better" were his words. We set the hour for an appointment.

As he entered the office he gripped my hand. "It was great. How do I look?"

I could hardly believe my eyes. Such demands on the physical and emotional strength would have drained the average pilot. . . . Not so with Peter. His face was smiles, his eyes clear, his voice strong. The full head of hair turning gray, plus an athletic body. . . . I'm sure he was taken for a movie star many times.

I said, "You look marvelous. If you feel as good as you look, you're over the top."

He sat down, then said, "I told my wife last night that I can sleep in any bed, so we're moving from one bed to another each week."

I laughed. "Feel free to sleep in any of the beds in your apartment [Central Park East], but in so doing, you must not get locked into the same pattern: Monday, east bedroom; Tuesday, west bedroom; etc."

"Sure . . . I never thought of that. But I'm able to sleep any damn place I please, at any time I become sleepy."

"The manner in which you have overcome the sickness is good. There are some people who with money have retired and allowed themselves to drift into a state of narcosis."

"That sounds worse than insomnia. . . . What does it mean?"

"It means this type of person handles the pain of neuroticism by sleeping fourteen or sixteen hours a day."

"Oh Lord, that will never happen to me. . . . I believe that sleep is necessary to stay alive . . . it's better not to be enslaved by the lack of it, or too much of it."

"Well said."

"Wife and I are going out on the town tonight. . . . I want to thank you for saving my life."

"Peter, this time, you can't thank me . . . the method I used with you is that of my friend Dr. Bryan Forrester, who passed away two years ago. I may never have the opportunity of using it again, but I'm glad it turned out well with you."

"I still want to thank you . . . you did it. What about your own bout with sleeplessness? Conquer it?"

"Yes, but not as thoroughly as you have. . . . Sleep means little to me; I learned that I can function on a high level with five or six hours of sleep. There are nights when sleep will not come. I'm delighted; I jump out of bed, grab a robe, and start doing all the things I love to do but don't have the opportunity of doing because of the hours I work."

"I think that's wonderful. . . . What do you do, say, if you go to sleep and wake up at three in the morning?"

"That's become my favorite time. I read books . . . books which I would never otherwise get to read. Then I write poetry; don't tell anybody because my poetry will never see printer's ink! Three o'clock in the morning is my favorite time to express myself in this manner. It is at that time I also write books and articles."

Before leaving he said, "I don't think I'll need your professional services ever again, but let's keep in touch."

We shook hands. "Let's keep in touch," I said.

He was a happy man. Less than two months prior to that last

visit to my office, he was in the hospital, a suicidal case with both wrists slashed.

Three years have gone by. Peter and I have kept in touch. But he seems now to be a person making up for the time he spent in the nerve-racking advertising business. He and his wife recently returned from a leisurely trip around the world. As they have no children of their own, he has set up a foundation for abandoned children in this country. He has done the same for children in Vietnam, Korea, the Philippines, and Bangladesh.

I do not have Peter's money, and I'm glad he's using it in a generous manner. However, the joy of helping a man like this means more than money can bring. There is a peace which the world cannot give, or take away. Working successfully with this desperate man reminds me that the deepest of satisfactions are found in a variety of unexpected places.

IX

The Stutterer Speaks

My secretary said, "You'll have to take the phone, I can't understand the man on the line."

I took the phone and I too could not understand him, but I immediately surmised what the situation was and what the man wanted. He could not pronounce his name, but I told him the free time I had for the following week. "How about Thursday at four?"

He grunted affirmatively. I gave him my address and hoped we had the few details clear.

It was an amazing experience for me to pick up the New York *Times*, December 15, 1974, and read a large headline on the front page, HYPNOTISM LEADS TO A HIT-RUN SUSPECT. The article began by saying, "The police have arrested a suspect in a hit-and-run accident after using hypnosis to help a policeman who witnessed the accident to recall part of the license-plate number of the car involved."

The story goes on to say that the policeman who saw the accident was taken to a physician who hypnotized him and was able to extract from his memory several letters of the license plate. The suspect in the case was thus caught and arrested. Why do I say I was amazed to see this story in headlines in the *Times?* For the reason that the *Times* allocates space according to quotas determined by importance. For instance, in the obituary column, there is a stated policy on how much space is to be given and whether or not a picture should be used with the story of one who has died. Were the editors surprised and impressed that a person's memory could be sharpened so that recalling the number on a license plate could be accomplished by hypnosis? To those of us who work in this field every day, this appears to be confusing a flea with an elephant. Such

memory recall is an infinitesimal feat compared to working successfully with certain other subjects—the stutterer, for instance. When
the stutterer reaches adulthood, his chances of ever speaking
fluently are extremely low. He may attend remedial-reading classes,
or remedial-speaking classes, he may see a physician or analyst—
and never be noticeably helped. I am convinced that the stutterer
stands a better chance of speech improvement through hypnosis
than by any other means. One of the obstacles the analyst has in
helping the severe stutterer is the time element. Within a fifty-
minute period the patient will say so little that the non-hypnotic
therapist becomes frustrated by the attempt to secure basic information.

He came in on the dot, Thursday at four. We shook hands, he attempted to say, "Glad to meet you." It was an ordeal for him to get
these words out. I asked him to be seated on the couch, and I began
the conversation by asking his name. He attempted, as he had done
on the phone, to speak his name. What came out was quite unin-
telligible. I was impressed with his immaculate dress and handsome
appearance. He was a black man whom I took to be about thirty
years of age, tall with a muscular frame. I then began to explain
that I would make every effort to assist him. His nerves loosened a
bit, he smiled and nodded his head. I told him that I was first of all
interested in putting him in a hypnotic state of relaxation and to
discover whether or not under hypnosis he could speak freely. He
liked that; that's why he came to me. He did not want any additional probing questions, which, because of his impediment, he had
great difficulty in answering, and coming to a minister, he was not
interested in a sermon or a prayer.

"Sit quietly, be as comfortable as possible, close your eyes for
about sixty seconds."

He paused, and I continued, "Keep eyes closed . . . now five
deep breaths . . . relaxation will become increasingly noticeable
with each breath."

At the end of the fifth breath his head went toward the chin, eyes
began to flutter. Then I said, "Your head will become heavier and
heavier . . . let it move to the right, to the left, or toward the chest
. . . do not let it move backward. Let your eyelids become as heavy
as they wish to become . . . as heavy as *they* wish to become."

As I asked him to enter the "breathing of sleep," I knew he was a responsive subject . . . muscles in the face, particularly across the forehead and around the jaw, were relaxed, his hands had grown heavy, he stretched his legs out in a position of peace and comfort. By the time I gave the suggestion of being drowsy and sleepy, the subconscious had emerged.

I then said, "At this point, if I said your right hand will levitate until it touches your face, the hand would move upward; if I said your hand would be cold, it would become cold, or hot, it would become hot . . . but I will suggest none of these things. I want you to talk to me . . . take it easy and take your time."

I paused for several seconds, thinking, "Would he or wouldn't he?"

"What is your full name?"

His reply in a beautiful baritone voice, perfect diction and controlled volume, "Roosevelt Wilson Jones."

"How old are you?"

"I am thirty-two years old."

"What kind of work do you do?"

"My brother and I own a small grocery store in Harlem. . . . I go to school at night."

"High school?"

"No, college, City College of New York." He pronounced each word slowly and carefully.

"What is your major?"

"I am pre-law . . . I want to be a lawyer. Next year I graduate. . . . It took me eight years. . . ."

"Where would you like to study law?"

"Columbia University."

I said, "Roosevelt, you have covered quite a bit of ground for one day. . . . Your pronunciation and diction are perfect. I now suggest that when you come out of this trance you will speak clearly and at our next session we will continue the conversation in the same relaxed manner. . . . Do you understand?"

"I understand," he said with confidence, still under hypnosis.

His mind cleared immediately. I waited for him to speak first. Waiting was interminable. At last he tried to say, "Thank you." It came out haltingly between gasps of breath.

I said to him, "Can you tell me your name?"

He half smiled. "Roosevelt Wilson Jones." This too was halting but with no gasping for breath.

"See you tomorrow, same time?"

He nodded. We shook hands and he left. If I have ever agreed to take a person where I felt a compulsion to be of assistance, it was with this bright young man.

The next session went well. He had been unable to speak since early childhood. His parents died before he was fifteen years of age. His brother, the only other child in the family, was ten years older. Apparently a good businessman, he took Roosevelt at age twenty-one as a partner. Their business grew rapidly. The brother was married, two children. Roosevelt was not married but said under hypnosis, "I like the girls."

The posthypnotic session went much like the first one: "Your mind will be bright and clear, coordination between mental processes and speech will be perfect. You will pronounce your name without halting, without stuttering . . . easily and clearly you will speak your name."

Out of the trance, he looked at me and smiled, and said, "You want me to speak my name." One who listens to a stutterer often makes the mistake of helping with a word or sentence. When a word will not come forth and the afflicted one struggles for breath, it is almost more than the listener can do to sit still while he struggles. I had worked many times with stutterers but none so bad as Roosevelt, and I was determined not to break into a word or sentence.

"Yes, I want you to speak your name."

Out of the hypnotic trance, what came forth was worse than the day before. He could not pronounce his first name. He finally gave up. I said, "Try to pronounce your last name."

This he did, but with considerable effort.

I was determined not to give up. I asked him, "Do you wish to continue the hypnotic sessions?"

He nodded.

I did not realize how much encouragement he had received. Under hypnosis the subject not only hears the therapist but he hears himself when he speaks. Never before had he heard himself speak easily and clearly. The sound of his voice, the way he spoke the words under hypnosis was a thrill to him.

Roosevelt Wilson Jones has the distinction of being under my care longer than any other person: one full year, an average of two sessions a week. Both of us were bulldog determined.

At the end of the fifth week, his improvement in saying short sentences and in pronouncing his name, when *not* under hypnosis, was noticeable. He was excited and proud. At this point, I wondered how far hypnosis would take him. I had no way of knowing that he would progress any further than where he was at the moment.

Roosevelt had a church background and was somewhat acquainted with the Bible. At the end of the sixth session, I gave him a specific posthypnotic suggestion: "Your mind will be clear, your speech will be strong, and the diction perfect. When you are brought out of this trance, you will read from the Bible the 100th Psalm. The Bible is on the table next to you. It is open to the 100th Psalm." He came out of the trance with a determined look on his face. He reached for the Bible.

I cautioned him, "Take your time, read slowly, and if possible let the voice go into a lower register."

He nodded and then began to read:

> Make a joyful noise to the Lord, all the lands!
> Serve the Lord with gladness!
> Come into his presence with singing!
> Know that the Lord is God!
> It is he that made us, and we are his;
> We are his people, and the sheep of his pasture.
> Enter his gates with thanksgiving,
> And his courts with praise!
> Give thanks to him, bless his name!
> For the Lord is good;
> His steadfast love endures for ever,
> And his faithfulness to all generations.

Still being somewhat under the influence of the trance, he read these words slowly and deliberately. He halted several times, but he read this beautiful poem without struggling for breath or words.

He put the Bible on the table and said, "I can do it, I know I can do it."

"Every day this week, morning and night, get by yourself and read the 100th Psalm aloud. Experiment with higher and lower registers of the voice . . . pick out a tune and sing the words as well as read them. . . . Do you have a Bible at your apartment?" I asked.

"Yes," he said positively.

At the next session we attempted a conversation prior to hypnotic induction. It was slow and painful. Finally, I asked Roosevelt to read the Psalm as he had done morning and night since the last session. He attempted to read it but could not get through it. I asked him to sing it . . . any tune in a singing, chanting voice. This he did perfectly.

Deep into the trance I gave the posthypnotic suggestion: "You will read slowly and clearly the 100th Psalm when you are brought out of the trance."

At the count of five his eyes opened, the trance lessened, but was still with him. He read the Psalm perfectly. Then I gave him a new chapter of the Bible for his homework: I Corinthians 13, the Poem of Love. The words read as follows:

If I speak in the tongues of men and of angels, but have not love, I am a noisy gong or a clanging cymbal. And if I have prophetic power, and understand all mysteries and all knowledge, and if I have all faith, so as to remove mountains, but have not love, I am nothing. If I give away all I have, and if I deliver my body to be burned, but have not love, I gain nothing.

Love is patient and kind; love is not jealous or boastful; it is not arrogant or rude. Love does not insist on its own way; it is not irritable or resentful; it does not rejoice at wrong, but rejoices in the right. Love bears all things, believes all things, hopes all things, endures all things.

Love never ends; as for prophecy, it will pass away; as for tongues, they will cease; as for knowledge, it will pass away. For our knowledge is imperfect and our prophecy is imperfect; but when the perfect comes, the imperfect will pass away. When I was a child, I spoke like a child, I thought like a child, I reasoned like a child; when I became a man, I gave up childish ways. For now we see in a mirror dimly, but then face to face. Now I know in part; then I shall understand fully, even as I have been fully understood. So faith, hope, love abide, these three; but the greatest of these is love.

I then read the Love Poem aloud. He listened intently to these magnificent words which he had not heard since he was a child.

I was able to understand him when he said, "When I was a small boy my mother used to read that part of the Bible to me."

I said, "I'm delighted you're familiar with it. That section will be your homework the next two weeks; read it aloud, each morning and night, alone. Take it slowly. If you get hung up, move on to the next word."

After two weeks with the "greatest love poem ever written," there was a decided improvement in Roosevelt's speech. . . . He knew it, I knew it. One day, he came in. Without any small talk I asked him to read for me the Love Poem. He took the Bible, found the place, and read without the assistance of hypnosis each word without halting or struggling.

"That's great," I exclaimed. "Now we are going to do something that will challenge you." I took him into my church sanctuary, to the pulpit, and said, "I'll sit in the back of the church. You stand in the pulpit and read from the Bible precisely as you read in the counseling room."

I went to the rear of the church. Roosevelt began to read. Few speakers are blessed with such rich quality of voice. I listened both fascinated and thrilled. He completed the reading; we went back into the counseling room.

I said, "Roosevelt, we have completed the hypnotic sessions. . . . From here on, you will come in as you have for the past seven or eight months and we'll just talk. I'll expect you to carry the conversation."

Then I asked him an important question, "How are you doing at the store with customers and what about your fellow students?"

He replied, "Those I know, I have no trouble with . . . with strangers . . ." Then he laughed. "However, my greatest stumbling block is the telephone. . . . I get hung up there."

"Make an effort the next few weeks to talk to strangers. Go out of your way to do it . . . the telephone will take care of itself."

For the next several weeks in our non-hypnotic sessions we talked mainly about those areas where he was still having difficulty. He wanted to be with young women. He wanted to date. For his homework the next week, he would seek out a woman to whom he was attracted, and ask her for a date to the movies or to one of the great museums which grace our city. He grinned and said, "I've already done it. . . . I was saving that for a surprise to you." Then he paused and said, "Her name is Irma . . . and she likes me."

I said, "So you're ahead of me. . . . I'll give you another assignment. In my Sunday service I have a lay person read the Scripture lesson for the morning. . . . Week after next Sunday, I want you, Roosevelt Wilson Jones, to be my assistant in the service. I want you to read to the congregation the Love Poem." Up to the present, there was nothing that I asked him to do which he resisted. He hesitated for a long time.

Then he said, "I'll do it."

"Saturday, come in. I'll go to the back of the church as before and you will go to the pulpit and read."

On this assignment we shook hands.

Saturday of the following week arrived. He went to the pulpit, I to the rear of the church. He read . . . magnificently, he read. No halting, no gasping, no hyperventilation; naturally, easily, putting meaning into the words, Roosevelt read the Love Poem. Never before had he been to my Sunday service. He did not know the people; the people did not know him. Members of the congregation assumed he was a ministerial student from one of the local seminaries. All were impressed with his appearance, his natural manner, but most of all with the resonance and control of voice.

One member of my official board, after learning that the reader of the morning was not a ministerial student, made a prophetic statement: "If that young man is not studying for the ministry—he should be."

Roosevelt Wilson Jones changed his mind about becoming a lawyer. He graduated from New York's Union Theological Seminary in the early 1970s and has been an active pastor in upper New York State since that time.

X

The Future of Hypnosis

History has its ups and downs; generations delight in *accepting* faiths and practices rejected by their elders or *rejecting* faiths and practices held sacred by their elders. Hypnosis has been a swing phenomenon for many years in many countries of the world. Currently, it is in public demand in Japan, England, the Soviet Union, and many other European countries. Our people, on the other hand, have never been, to any great extent, open to it, but rather have been suspicious of hypnosis since its inception. This in spite of the fact that a host of prominent names have been associated with it. Names of men whose scholarship and scientific integrity have been unquestioned. Yet this has not changed the minds of people in business and industry, of medical schools, of seminaries and churches, and of the people who staff our colleges.

Reasons for this resistance are not easy to come by. Is it possible that the "danger" in hypnosis has been emphasized out of proportion? In all of the years I have been into hypnosis both as a practitioner and in research, not *one* person has ever had an adverse experience. Some may not have been helped as much as they would like, but none have been injured in any way. Is it possible that the stage and nightclub performers have turned people away? Is it possible that American people equate hypnosis with "spiritualism" or even with the more weird aspects of the occult? Of course, there is some truth in all this, but a logical answer eludes us at this particular time. Ordinarily, American people do not turn away from a phenomenon just because it is dangerous or because it has been witnessed in a nightclub or because it may be associated with the occult.

In the first chapter I related how my friend Professor John

Handy spoke sharply to me when I insisted that a man as great as Sigmund Freud tried hypnosis and gave it up because it would not work. Of course, I have since learned that this misunderstanding has been handed down, so that today in many academic circles the same opinion about Freud and hypnosis is held. Though in his work with neurotics he preferred "free association," Freud not only retained a respect for hypnosis through his lifetime, but also went deeper and deeper into the subject we now call parapsychology. Freud wrote to a friend:

> The strongest literary impression of this month came to me from a report on telepathy experiments with Professor Gilbert Murray from the *Proceedings* of the Society for Psychical Research, December, 1924. I confess that the impression made by these reports was so strong that I am ready to give up my opposition to the existence of thought-transference. I should even be prepared to lend the support of psychoanalysis to the matter of telepathy.

Freud further wrote:

> I am now far from willing to repudiate without further ado all these phenomena, concerning which we possess so many minute observations even from men of intellectual prominence, and which should certainly form a basis for further investigation. We may even hope that some of these observations will be explained by our nascent knowledge of the unconscious psychic processes, without necessitating radical changes in our present outlook.

At the moment the future of hypnosis hangs in the balance in various areas of American life. It can go in either direction, toward greater oblivion and misunderstanding or toward a responsible place in the healing professions.

At this time, I refuse to be as pessimistic as Dr. G. H. Estabrooks, who in his splendid book *Hypnosis* wrote the following:

> It is very difficult for the average reader to realize how strong this power of prejudice [towards hypnosis] may be. The writer has a friend, one of the great psychiatrists of the country, a

former president of the American Psychiatric Association. This man made the statement that even if he were convinced of the value of hypnotism in treating nervous disorders he would not dare use it in his institution, one of the country's best state hospitals for nervous diseases. There would be too many unpleasant questions to be answered!

Yet this particular doctor is well known for courage and for broad-mindedness.

There is not one member of the medical profession in either Utica or Syracuse, to mention specific cities, who uses hypnotism in his practice. Why? Popular prejudice, nothing more. . . . The stage hypnotist, the "professional," has so disgusted the average citizen with his exhibitions that it will be many years before hypnosis will regain the prestige which it now enjoys in Europe, where such shows are illegal.

1. Business and Industry

Sam Church sat in my counseling room, looked straight toward me, and said, "Remember me?"

"Of course I remember you. Your name is Sam Church and you completed a series of ten sessions with me the first part of last year." (I had checked the name with my secretary before he came in.)

"That's right. . . . Do you recall my work?"

"You're in the brokerage business, or . . ."

"Dead wrong."

Then I said quickly, "You're an insurance salesman."

"I guess you would call me an insurance salesman. . . . I am executive vice-president of the —— Insurance Company. At the time I came to see you I preferred to be listed as 'insurance salesman.'"

Mr. Church, short and bald, was about sixty years of age. He dressed conservatively and spoke fluently with a pleasant voice. I remembered that he came to me for hypnosis with fewer problems than anyone I had recently seen. "All I want," he had said, "is to find a way to relax . . . my blood pressure is a little high and I despise taking pills . . . never been sick a day in my life. One of our salesmen saw you two years ago . . . blocked memory, not an ounce of concentration. You helped him; I thought you might do the same for me."

Sam Church had been easy to work with. Following the first session he exclaimed, "What a marvelous sensation. . . . I feel loose and limber. . . . I heard you most of the time, but can't remember everything you said. . . . I was too busy drifting and floating around the planets." Sam thought it was a miracle that he could become relaxed but especially that his blood pressure could be brought down by becoming loose, less tense. He could not get over it. He kept saying, "It's a miracle, a real miracle."

Now, one year later, he looked at me with a twinkle in his eye and said, "I'm here to offer you a job, a full-time job. I don't know what your present salary is, but . . ."

He knew my salary was not very high. I was listening intently.

He continued, "Since I came to see you, I've been talking to several men in the company about the proposal I now make. They agree with me that our company should have someone with knowledge and skills to be our full-time resident in hypnosis."

Mr. Church was loquacious. An article in the New York *Post,* December 21, 1974, brought the decision to a head. The company would save a great deal of money if its employees had easy access to such services. (The number of employees is in the thousands.) This article, written by Marsha Kranes, described how famous attorney F. Lee Bailey employed hypnosis in criminal cases. I read the article and filed it. I especially appreciated Bailey's quote concerning his use of hypnosis: "You can get the truth or bizarre fantasy; you can't always tell the difference. But it's a very rapid way of getting inside the head of the accused. Primarily it is a way of getting information that can later be checked out and developed."

Marsha Kranes quoted Dr. Milton V. Kline, Manhattan psychiatrist, who said that he was asked to hypnotize an emotionally disturbed ten-year-old girl who had been sexually molested. She was unable to remember the crime until she was hypnotized. Kline said, "Then she recalled everything," and was able to provide information that led investigators to a suspect and the development of other evidence. The Japanese, according to Dr. Kline, have made impressive advances in this area and have established institutes for rehabilitation through hypnosis at two major universities. The article goes on to say that a prominent New York anesthesiologist claims 90 per cent success in using hypnosis for pain problems. He also uses hypnosis for a number of surgical procedures, including normal births and Caesarean sections.

So the article in the *Post* brought the matter to a head and also sent the vice-president of the company hurrying to my office.

Mr. Church continued: "Do you know how much money the company loses because of absenteeism? Of course you don't and there is no point in telling you except to say the figure is in the thousands . . . smokers with their ailments, alcoholics, listless and disinterested people, sex problems, phobias . . . I could go on and on." And I am sure he could!

"I'll get to the point. We'll pay you three times your present salary, provide you with a lovely counseling room, the company's fringe benefits will be yours, your position will be on a professional level. . . . We would like to have you begin within two months. What do you say? Or do you want a couple of days to think it over?"

I had been taken by surprise, but as Mr. Church talked, I knew precisely what my answer had to be. I said, "I do not need more time to think it over. . . . I appreciate your offer but . . ."

When I injected the word "but," his face fell. He had done some investigating, and was sure that I could not turn down the offer. Before he could say anything I continued, "Come back in two years, and we'll talk business."

"You mean that?"

"Yes, I mean it. . . . I have recommended this idea to several firms in various parts of the country. . . . Some companies will hire ministers as chaplains. I know of none that will hire one with a background in hypnosis. Your company is the first. I mean what I say. . . . If the offer is still open in two years, I will talk business with you." (Within two years from that date I will have completed forty years in the ministry.)

What now must hypnosis do, what more must it accomplish to get off the comedian's stage and become a respectable part of the healing professions? All over the world it is happening—the Soviet Union, England, Austria, Japan, the Scandinavian countries, and elsewhere. Sam Church was a businessman who when dealing with employees was not handing out welfare checks. Each employee had to earn *more* for the company than he was paid. When he offered me a position the same principle applied. I am sure he had thought through the number of employees I could see in one day, the approximate percentage that could be helped, and the amount of money his company would save by keeping more employees well and functioning.

As long as a company is fair with its employees, as is the case with Sam Church's, I see nothing wrong with this principle. The very least a firm, a company, a corporation could do at this time would be to appoint a high-level committee and study the matter relating to hypnosis from every angle. Such potential power for good should not be bypassed as if it did not exist.

There is a footnote to this emphasis concerning big business. I am a fan of all kinds of sports, especially professional baseball, football, basketball. It is impossible for me to understand the reluctance of any "pro" team to employ a consultant in hypnosis. A hitter in a slump tries every trick in the bag to break out . . . foot here, foot there, stance is changed, new grips are tried, lighter bats and heavier bats are used, coaches become as anxious as the hitter in the slump. I give the men in this form of big business a hint: no season should pass without these high-strung, gifted athletes having immediate access to the power of hypnosis.

2. Medical Schools

If the demand for help by hypnosis continues to grow in various parts of the world, more medical schools, including dental schools, will be forced to offer specific training in the field. They will do this for physicians, surgeons, psychiatrists, and dentists. It will be done as naturally as the study of anatomy or the art of using the knife. There are two types of doctors who may use hypnosis in their practice. The first, I abhor. He is the man with the M.D. degree who discovers that the public is now more receptive to the use of hypnosis than ever before. He reads a book or maybe two books and discards his practice of general medicine. He devotes his entire time to seeing patients—using nothing but hypnosis—and becomes known as a specialist! Result: his income quadruples within a year. He now charges a hundred dollars for thirty or forty minutes, no house calls, no hospital calls.

The second doctor or analyst, I admire. He senses that a great body of knowledge was omitted in his various studies in college and in medical or psychoanalytic school. At a late date in his practice he wants to incorporate hypnosis in his work. He reads, he attends conferences and special classes, and seeks assistance from those experienced in the field. His motive in doing this is not to make an extra dollar; he genuinely desires to be of more help to his patients.

This leads to the question of licensing people who intend to use hypnosis as a healing aid. How should this be done? For God's sake —and I use that term reverently—it should not be done according to a scholastic degree. The first doctor I mentioned possesses A.B., M.A., and M.D. degrees; he practiced medicine for twenty years totally ignorant of hypnosis—its history, theory, techniques of induction, and applications of its healing power. By reading two books, he becomes a specialist in hypnosis! Today, the average lay hypnotist knows more about hypnosis than this man will ever know. If the degree is not the determining factor, what then? Four rigid requirements should be expected of any individual who wishes to practice hypnosis: a 25,000-word paper setting forth his understanding of hypnosis; a comprehensive written test; an oral test conducted by a committee of men and women who are specialists in the field; he should also be required to give demonstrations of his skills before such a committee.

It is obvious to the reader that I am opposed to hypnosis being used as entertainment on stage, on television, or in a nightclub. An entertainer should not be able to perform simply by calling himself a "mentalist." The same goes for dozens of groups such as Mind Control, Mind Dynamics, Mind Expansion, E.S.T., etc., which have hypnosis as the modus operandi but up to this point are wary of using the word for fear they will get in trouble with the law or that they will turn off prospective customers.

3. Seminaries and Divinity Schools

Seminaries and divinity schools are theologically oriented, and each is expected to do the same thing. Until recently the difference in name was due to the divinity school being an integral part of a university, one of several graduate schools. The seminary was usually separate from university control and mainly prepared men for the parish ministry. Most of our "name" universities—such as Harvard, Princeton, Yale, Brown—began as theological schools.

I doubt that hypnosis will ever become *totally* acceptable in our country so long as the church and its seminaries refuse to approve it. This is a pity, for the reason that such schools have broadened the standard theological curriculum so that such subjects as social studies (man and his environment), psychology of religion (man and his inner life), and pastoral counseling (the minister as healer) are required for graduation. Pastoral counseling and clinical studies in mental hospitals have become so dominant in some theological schools that it has created a problem for certain members of the faculty who feel that the original courses in theology and the Bible are being de-emphasized and "fad" courses are being taught.

In my judgment, courses in the history, theory, and techniques of hypnosis could take the place of certain psychological courses which often appear to be neither religion nor psychology. At this time there is no seminary or divinity school in the country (or world) that teaches hypnosis to prospective clergymen. Several have launched into the waters of Zen Buddhism, transcendental meditation, and yoga, but not hypnosis.

It is possible that a pastoral counselor would not choose to use hypnosis even if he were trained in it, or it is possible that the occasion in a counseling situation would never arise when he felt any real need for it. But what about his own life? The weight of being the spiritual leader of a congregation, no matter the size, is indeed difficult and complicated. A person who knows what self-induction is may never be able to achieve results such as those he would receive by working with a specialist in the field. However, with self-induction there is a degree of relaxation which can be achieved.

There develops a greater ability to cope with a world which sometimes seems to have gone mad. Self-induction helps him to gain a more accurate knowledge of himself so that he becomes a stronger and more stable person.

Nearly twenty years ago I wrote a feature article for *Life* magazine which achieved national and international attention. It was entitled "Why Ministers Are Cracking Up." At that time in American history, men of God were not supposed to manifest any abnormal emotional symptoms; they were men of faith, God would do the rest. I do not question the power of faith in God, but I do know that God moves in mysterious ways His wonders to perform and that the gift of His presence is not limited to the man who rests his soul only upon conventional prayer. The *Life* article stirred the clergy, shook the church, and inspired seminaries and churches to examine their own programs as well as their expectations of ministers. I am hopeful that this book will shake seminaries and churches as did the *Life* article.

4. The College Campus

On a certain college campus there is a designated building to which students may retreat when they begin to feel they are "uptight" or perhaps at the breaking point. This building is not a church or chapel, it is a building where students learn to unwind by doing yoga breathing, sensitivity exercises in groups, meditation, or finding relief through chanting. Students under pressure are no different from other people under pressure; they begin to act in strange and often unacceptable ways; they experiment with marijuana or "coke" or perhaps even one of the harder drugs such as alcohol or heroin.

Why not hypnosis? Every college or university now has access to at least one psychiatrist whose specific job is to assist students in emotional or mental trouble. In my judgment, the administration should do one of two things in connection with the use of hypnosis. Either the therapist should be a psychiatrist trained in the process or he should be a highly qualified hypnotherapist who claims no psychiatric credentials.

Two years ago, I enjoyed a private conference with Frederick C. Munns, M.B.S.H., secretary of the British Society of Hypnotherapists. We were in his office in London tossing questions and answers to each other. At one point Mr. Munns said, "Hypnosis is more in demand in England than perhaps ever before. Many people have been sorely disappointed with *endless* years of psychotherapy; some have turned to the occult but many more are seeking help through hypnosis." I questioned him concerning the attitude of young people of college age and those in their thirties and was pleased and surprised to hear him say that the same interest existed as with older adults. However, many young people in England seek help from hypnosis only after they have experimented with certain aspects of the occult.

The only time we read or hear of a college student being helped by hypnosis is under extreme and most dramatic circumstances, some of which are in this book. Marsha Kranes, in the *Post* article previously referred to, describes the work of a hypnotist in Los Angeles by the name of Arthur Ellen. Ellen has worked miracles with such athletes as Ken Venturi, Orlando Cepeda, Richie Allen, and Maury Wills, as well as celebrities such as Tony Curtis and Fernando Lamas. In the future it would be gratifying if young people, under stress, had access to a specialist in hypnosis. It need not be a dramatic occasion; it could be the relief of anxiety and building confidence without drugs or alcohol!

There is hardly a man of letters of our time more prolific and more imaginative than Aldous Huxley. Huxley was deeply committed to the power of hypnosis. In the mammoth-size book, 991 pages, entitled *Letters of Aldous Huxley,* edited by Grover Smith, Huxley devotes considerable space, in more than thirty-five letters, to hypnosis and his experience with it. In a letter to a friend (July 20, 1952) he gives testimony to the power of hypnosis, especially in its anesthetic effects. He writes:

> I myself am not a particularly good hypnotic subject, but can go at least into a light trance. When I had my bout of iritis [inflammation of the iris] last year I went two or three times to a man who is head of the Psychology Department at the University of California at Los Angeles, and these brief hypnotic treat-

ments undoubtedly helped me to sleep and to deal with the pain. Moreover, by means of auto-hypnosis (which is an art not too hard to acquire if one has a good hypnotist as a teacher) and by treatments from Maria [Huxley's first wife] and our friend (Leslie) LeCron, the psycho-therapist, I was enabled to get over the very considerable apprehension which accompanied and followed the iritis—apprehension that the good eye might be involved and lose much of its vision, and apprehension of a relapse, which is not uncommon in these conditions.

In all these instances the benefits due to hypnosis are due fundamentally to the fact that it is accompanied by a high degree of relaxation, mental and physical. The ego is able to let go, to get out of the way, to stop interfering with the beneficent action of the "entelechy," which is at once the physiological sub-conscious that sees to the proper functioning of the body, and the higher, non-personal sub-conscious—the thing that, in contradistinction to the personal sub-conscious where the Freudian rats and black-beetles are active, gives one "inspirations," "intuitions," "good thoughts" which are as genuinely real facts as are the fears and compulsions, aggressions and despairs generated in the Freudian basement.

On the basis of what I myself have experienced, of what I have seen in the case of Maria, of what I have been able to accomplish in the case of several friends, of what I have seen done by LeCron and, more recently, by a man who is probably the greatest living virtuoso in the field of hypnosis, Dr. (———), I would advise you very strongly to try hypnosis. Since success depends on a satisfactory relation between the hypnotized person and the operator, you must be prepared to "shop around" until you find someone sympathetic as well as skilful.

What is the future of hypnosis in the various areas of our society? I predict the first breakthrough will come in industry and business. Strange as it may seem, the honest profit motive will make it so! When corporation executives discover the immeasurable potential for good in hypnosis as applied to their own lives as well as to their employees', tides of resistance will be broken so much that among professionally trained people there will be a hurried, and I hope a thorough, effort to supply the demand for competent hypnotists.

The next breakthrough will take place in medical schools; it may have already begun. Many of my personal friends, my age, in medicine and psychotherapy, are embarrassed that they could go through twenty or more years of formal study and not be introduced to a field of study which is more scientifically oriented than many subjects they were required to pass. Many of these men are now making up for lost time by a discipline of serious study of the history, theory, techniques, and applications of hypnotic power.

Next, the college campus. The beginning of the demand here will likely take place in athletic departments! Nowhere else can an "uptight" athlete acquire and maintain a clear, bright mind in a relaxed body. A tranquilizer tranquilizes both body and mind. Neither alcohol, drugs, nor the knife can produce genuine tranquility while at the same time keeping the body strong and the mind alert. Hypnosis can.

Last and least, alas, are the churches and seminaries. These institutions for years to come will continue to prefer that their spiritually endowed men go into the military, into industry, and into the pulpit equipped to pray, preach, and counsel in conventional ways. For the church to consider the amazing power of hypnosis as an extension of the power of God is just too much.

In the area of churches and seminaries, therefore, I share Dr. Estabrooks' pessimism (quoted in this chapter). However, in the healing professions it is possible that in our time we shall see a significant increase in the use of hypnosis as an aid toward relieving human suffering.

SUGGESTED READING

Adler, Alfred. *Understanding Human Nature.* Garden City, N.Y.: Garden City Publishing Company, 1927.

Baudouin, C. *Suggestion and Autosuggestion.* New York: Dodd, Mead & Company, 1922.

Bramwell, J. M. *Hypnotism: Its History, Practice and Theory.* Philadelphia: J. B. Lippincott Company, 1903.

Breuer, J., and Freud, S. *Studies in Hysteria.* Nervous and Mental Disease Monograph Series, 1936.

Brill, A. A. (ed.). *The Basic Writings of Sigmund Freud.* New York: The Modern Library, 1938.

Brown, W. *Psychology and Psychotherapy.* London: Edward Arnold & Co., 1934.

Burgess, Anthony. *A Clockwork Orange.* New York: Ballantine Books, 1962.

Cayce, Edgar Evans, and Cayce, Hugh Lynn. *The Outer Limits of Edgar Cayce's Power.* New York: Harper & Row, 1971.

Davis, L. W., and Husband, R. W. "A Study of Hypnotic Susceptibility in Relation to Personality Traits," *Journal of Abnormal and Social Psychology,* 26: 175–82, 1931.

Estabrooks, G. H. *Hypnotism.* New York: E. P. Dutton & Co., 1943.

Forel, A. *Hypnotism.* New York: Allied Publications, 1927.

Fromm, Erica, and Shor, Ronald E. (eds.). *Research Developments and Perspectives.* New York: Aldine-Atherton, 1972.

Fromm, Erich. *Psychoanalysis and Religion.* New Haven: Yale University Press, 1950.

———. *The Art of Loving.* New York: Harper & Row, 1956.

Haley, Jay. *Uncommon Therapy: Therapy through Hypnotic Dynamics.* New York: Ballantine Books, 1973. (This book is a description of the psychiatric techniques of Milton H. Erickson, M.D.)

Heron, L. T. *ESP in the Bible.* New York: Doubleday & Company, 1974.

Hollander, B. *Methods and Uses of Hypnosis and Self-Hypnosis.* London: George Allen & Unwin, 1935.

Hull, C. L. *Hypnosis and Suggestibility.* New York: D. Appleton-Century, 1933.

188   THE AMAZING POWER OF HYPNOSIS

Jung, C. G. *Modern Man in Search of a Soul.* New York: Harcourt, Brace & Company, 1933.

———. *Psychology and Religion.* New Haven: Yale University Press, 1938.

Karlins, Marvin, and Andrews, Lewis M. *Biofeedback.* Philadelphia: J. B. Lippincott Company, 1972.

LeCron, L. M. *The Complete Guide to Hypnosis.* Los Angeles: Nash Publishing Corporation, 1971.

——— and Bordeaux, J. *Hypnotism Today.* New York: Grune & Stratton, 1947.

Lindner, R. M. *Rebel Without a Cause.* New York: Grune & Stratton, 1944.

Luce, Gay Gaer, and Segal, Julius. *Sleep.* New York: Lancer Books, 1966.

——— and ———. *Insomnia.* New York: Doubleday & Company, 1969.

Mahararishi Mahesh Yogi. *Transcendental Meditation.* New York: New American Library, 1968.

Marks, R. W. *The Story of Hypnotism.* New York: Prentice-Hall, 1947.

May, Rollo. *Love and Will.* New York: W. W. Norton & Company, 1969.

Mears, Ainslie. *A System of Medical Hypnosis.* New York: Julian Press, 1960.

Metzner, Ralph. *Maps of Consciousness.* New York: The Macmillan Company, 1971.

Pines, Maya. *The Brain Changers.* New York: Harcourt Brace Jovanovich, 1973.

Prince, M. *The Unconscious.* New York: The Macmillan Company, 1929.

Rhodes, Raphael. *Hypnosis: Theory, Practice and Application.* New York: Citadel Press, 1950.

Satow, L. *Hypnotism and Suggestion.* New York: Dodd, Mead & Company, 1923.

Sidis, B. *An Experimental Study of Sleep.* Boston: Richard G. Badger, 1909.

Skinner, B. F. *Beyond Freedom and Dignity.* New York: Alfred A. Knopf, 1971.

Stern, Jess. *The Search for a Soul: Taylor Caldwell's Psychic Lives.* New York: Doubleday & Company; Fawcett Crest Book, 1972.

Sugrue, Thomas. *The Story of Edgar Cayce.* New York: Dell Publishing Co., 1942.

Tart, Charles T. (ed.). *Altered States of Consciousness.* New York: Doubleday Anchor Book, 1972.

Weatherhead, Leslie D. *Psychology, Religion and Healing.* New York: Abingdon Press, 1941.

Wetterstrand, O. G. *Hypnotism and Its Application to Practical Medicine.* New York: G. P. Putnam's Sons, 1902.

Wolberg, Lewis R. *Hypnoanalysis.* New York: Grune & Stratton, 1945.

———. *Hypnosis: Is It for You?* New York: Harcourt Brace Jovanovich, 1972.

Wolpe, Joseph. *The Practice of Behavior Therapy.* New York: Pergamon Press, 1969.